Selective Digestive Tract Decontamination in Intensive Care Medicine: a Practical Guide to Controlling Infection

Peter H.J. van der Voort • Hendrick K.F. van Saene
Editors

Selective Digestive Tract Decontamination in Intensive Care Medicine: a Practical Guide to Controlling Infection

Springer

Peter H.J. van der Voort
Internist-intensivist
Department of Intensive Care
Onze Lieve Vrouwe Gasthuis
Amsterdam,
The Netherlands
p.voort3@chello.nl

Hendrick K.F. van Saene
Department of Clinical Microbiology
and Infection Control
Royal Liverpool Children's NHS
Trust of Alder Hey
Liverpool,
United Kingdom
Rick.VanSaene@RLC.NHS.UK

Cover illustration: it summarizes infection prevention in the intensive care.
Adapted by H.K.F. van Saene and reprinted with permission from: C.P. Stoutenbeek (1987) Infection prevention in intensive care. Infection prevention in multiple trauma patients by selective decontamination of the digestive tract (SDD). PhD thesis, Groningen

Library of Congress Control Number: 2007931632

ISBN 978-88-470-0652-2 Springer Milan Berlin Heidelberg New York
ISBN 978-88-470-0653-9 (eBook)

Springer is a part of Springer Science+Business Media
springer.com

Cover design: Simona Colombo, Milan, Italy
Typesetting: Graphostudio, Milan, Italy

Springer-Verlag Italia S.r.l., Via Decembrio 28, I-20137 Milan

Preface

Infection control in intensive care units is a continuing challenge. Since 1984, intensivists trying to prevent infection have had the option of applying a well-balanced and thoroughly studied approach called selective decontamination of the digestive tract (SDD). Over 20 years of clinical SDD research, 56 randomised controlled trials and 10 meta-analyses have been published. The effect on mortality is debated; the effect on infection control is not. SDD is not a costly manoeuvre. Resistance does not appear to be a clinical problem. Moreover, a growing body of evidence shows that SDD might be the method that could be used to control the worldwide emergence of resistant micro-organisms. However, SDD will not have these potential effects if healthcare professionals do not apply the philosophy properly and consistently. In addition, basic intensive care still needs to be adequate and the results of the cultures should be quickly and readily available. Doctors should be eager to get the results and to adjust their treatment accordingly. The effects of SDD can be completely lost in a multicentre study if these basic conditions are not all equally in place.

Many ICU physicians have questions about the practical implementation and application of SDD. In addition, it has been shown that the results obtained by individual ICUs vary in the degree of success in decontamination and the outcomes they reflect. A proper understanding of the principles and meticulous implementation in clinical practice will benefit patients and reduce both staff workloads and cost. These facts encouraged us to complete this volume on the principles and practice of SDD so as to provide a practical guide that can be used in daily decision-making on infection control. All the authors have been working with SDD in critically ill patients for many years. Their purpose in writing their chapters has been to share their knowledge with readers. Both healthcare workers who are about to start working with SDD in clinical practice and those who have already been working with SDD for some time but want to improve their practice can learn from these authors.

September 2007

Peter van der Voort
Hendrick K.F. van Saene

Contents

Contributors

Hans L. Bams, MD
Anaesthesiologist-intensivist, Skills Centre, University Hospital Groningen, Groningen, The Netherlands

Rik T. Gerritsen, MD
Internist-intensivist, Department of Intensive Care, Medical Centre Leeuwarden Leeuwarden, The Netherlands

Evert de Jonge, MD, PhD
Internist-intensivist, Department of Intensive Care, Academic Medical Centre Amsterdam, The Netherlands

Dave M. Mackie, MD, PhD
Anaesthesiologist-intensivist, Department of Anaesthetics, Intensive Care and Burns Unit, Red Cross Hospital
Beverwijk, The Netherlands

Jeanine Mysliwietz, RN
Intensive care nurse, Department of Intensive Care, Medical Centre Leeuwarden Leeuwarden, The Netherlands

Jetske Oenema, RN
Intensive care nurse, Department of Intensive Care, Medical Centre Leeuwarden Leeuwarden, The Netherlands

Heleen M. Oudemans-van Straaten, MD, PhD
Internist-intensivist, Department of Intensive Care, Onze Lieve Vrouwe Gasthuis Amsterdam, The Netherlands

Hans J. Rommes, MD, PhD
Internist-intensivist, Department of Intensive Care, Gelre Ziekenhuizen, Lukas Location
Apeldoorn, The Netherlands

Hendrick K.F. van Saene, MD, PhD
Department of Clinical Microbiology and Infection Control, Royal Liverpool Children's NHS Trust of Alder Hey
Liverpool, United Kingdom

Rients Schootstra, PharmD
Hospital pharmacist, Pharma Assist
Hoogeveen, The Netherlands

Markus J. Schultz, MD, PhD
Internist-intensivist, Department of Intensive Care, Academic Medical Centre
Amsterdam, The Netherlands

Hans I. van der Spoel, MD
Intensivist, Department of Intensive Care, Onze Lieve Vrouwe Gasthuis
Amsterdam, The Netherlands

Peter E. Spronk, MD, PhD
Internist-intensivist, Department of Intensive Care, Gelre Ziekenhuizen, Lucas Location
Apeldoorn, The Netherlands

Jacqueline E.H.M. Vet, MD
Anaesthesiologist-intensivist, Department of Anaesthesia, Intensive Care and Burns Unit, Red Cross Hospital
Beverwijk, The Netherlands

Peter H.J. van der Voort, MD, PhD, MSc
Internist-intensivist, Department of Intensive Care, Onze Lieve Vrouwe Gasthuis
Amsterdam, The Netherlands

Jan P. Yska, PharmD
Hospital Pharmacist, Department of Hospital Pharmacy, Medical Centre Leeuwarden
Leeuwarden, The Netherlands

Durk F. Zandstra, MD, PhD
Anaesthesiologist-Intensivist, Department of Intensive Care, Onze Lieve Vrouwe Gasthuis
Amsterdam, The Netherlands

List of Abbreviations

AGNB	Aerobic Gram-Negative Bacteria
APACHE	Acute Physiology and Chronic Health Evaluation
AR	Antimicrobial Resistance
BSI	Blood Stream Infection
C	Control
CAP	Community-Acquired Pneumonia
CFU	Colony Forming Units
COPD	Chronic Obstructive Pulmonary Disease
EBM	Evidence-Based Medicine
GALT	Gut-Associated Lymphoid Tissue
GCLP	Good Control Laboratory Practice
GMP	Good Manufacturing Practice
HAP	Hospital-Acquired Pneumonia
ICU	Intensive Care Unit
IgA	Immunoglobulin A
IPI	Intrinsic Pathogenicity Index
MIC	Minimal Inhibitory Concentration
MRAb	Multi-Resistant *Acinetobacter baumannii*
MRSA	Methicillin- or Multi-Resistant *Staphylococcus aureus*
NA	Not Available
OA	Ofloxacin - Amphotericin B
P	Placebo
PGA	Polymyxin - Gentamycin - Amphotericin B
PGN	Polymyxin - Gentamycin - Neomycin
PPM	Potentially Pathogenic Microorganism
PTA	Polymyxin E – Tobramycin – Amphotericin B
RCT	Randomised Controlled Trial
SAPS	Simplified Acute Physiology Score
SDD	Selective Digestive Tract Decontamination
SOD	Selective Oral Decontamination
TBSA	Total Burnt Skin Area
UTI	Urinary Tract Infection
VAP	Ventilator-Associated Pneumonia

Chapter 1
The History of Selective Decontamination of the Digestive Tract

Hendrick K.F. van Saene, Hans J. Rommes and Durk F. Zandstra

Introduction

In the 1950s the scope of the infection problem in hospitals changed. The introduction and widespread use of chemotherapeutic and antibiotic agents resulted in profound changes in the character of infections and microorganisms that were encountered. Deaths from community-acquired infection with gram-positive pathogens such as *S. pneumoniae, S. pyogenes* and *S. aureus* became less common, while the proportion of deaths attributable to hospital-acquired infections with aerobic gram-negative bacilli (AGNB) became manifest. These so-called nosocomial infections became increasingly prevalent in that period, especially in patients whose severe underlying disease was ameliorated by improving medical therapy. Infections due to AGNB became a frequent cause of death in patients treated for leukaemia or non-Hodgkin lymphoma, renal transplantation patients and patients on mechanical ventilation. In the 1960s and 1970s the frequency of nosocomial infections continued to be a problem despite the introduction of new broad-spectrum antibiotics. It became evident that it was not hospitalisation in itself that predisposed patients to infection; rather, the hospitalised patient was an "altered host" with enhanced susceptibility to infection. Feingold [1], in 1970, described two main reasons for higher susceptibility to infection: conditions impairing cellular or humoral defence mechanisms against infection, such as leukopenia, defective function of leucocytes, Hodgkin's disease and immunosuppressive therapy, and conditions compromising the mechanical defence barriers such as urinary and intravenous catheters, surgical wounds, burns and tracheostomy.

Another rapidly evolving problem was the emergence of antibiotic-resistant AGNB. The addition of a new antibiotic drug to the therapeutic arsenal invariably led to the emergence of resistant strains within a couple of years. In particular, *Pseudomonas aeruginosa*, which had become resistant to the available antibiotics was responsible for severe and often lethal nosocomial infections. Not surprisingly, the intensive care unit (ICU) was the single largest source of nosocomial infection in all hospitals in the 1960s and 1970s. Clustering of

P.H.J. van der Voort, H.K.F. van Saene (eds.) *Selective Digestive Tract Decontamination in Intensive Care Medicine.* © Springer 2008

patients with lowered defence against infection owing to their critical illness, use of invasive techniques for monitoring and life support, presence of many patients with infections and understaffing in often very busy units were factors contributing to high rates of nosocomial infections in intensive care units. In ICUs all over the world the emergence of infections caused by multi-resistant AGNB became an increasing problem. The wide-scale use of parenteral broad-spectrum antibiotics was responsible for selecting multiple resistant AGNB in the ICU. In the face of an increasing problem with infection and resistance, there was a reawakening of interest in the control of hospital-acquired, and more specifically ICU-acquired, infections. Epidemiologists found associations between nosocomial infections and a wide variety of predisposing factors, such as corticosteroids, indwelling urinary and venous catheters, mechanical ventilators, tracheostomies, broad-spectrum antibiotics and intravenous preparations. These studies led to numerous hospital procedures manuals replete with measures to prevent the transmission of microorganisms. Unfortunately, only a few of these procedures were clearly shown to lower the incidence of infection. Infection prevention specialists and microbiologists developed guidelines aimed at prevention of acquisition and subsequent carrying, and also at the emergence of resistant strains. Adherence to strict hygiene should control the transmission of microorganisms via the hands of healthcare workers. Five infection control manoeuvres, i.e., hand disinfection, isolation, personal protective equipment (gloves, gowns and aprons), care of patient's equipment and care of the environment should reduce the number of nosocomial infections. To prevent antimicrobial resistance, antimicrobials should not be given until after the infection has been diagnosed. These measures seem to have been unsuccessful for various reasons, being expensive, impractical in busy units, cumbersome and –very important– lacking a convincing effect on the incidence of infection. For example, Eickhoff and Daschner found a overall infection rate as high as 38% in surgical ICUs [2, 3], in contrast to the 5–10% rate of nosocomial infection in general wards. In 1974, Northey found a linear relationship between the duration of stay in the ICU and the infection rate [4]. In patients who were hit by such a severe illness that they needed more than 5 days of intensive care treatment the infection rate was as high as 80–90%. Fry, and two years later Goris, evaluated the impact of the infection problem on mortality [5, 6]. Both studies revealed that 80% of the late mortality in ICU patients was related to ICU-acquired infections. In multiple trauma patients the devastating effects of infection were particularly apparent. Previously healthy young people involved in an accident initially survived the trauma-related injury thanks to sophisticated life support techniques. However, a substantial number of them eventually died of ICU-acquired infection-related multiple organ failure after several weeks of intensive care treatment.

Surveillance cultures of throat and rectum uniquely detect the carrier state, whether it be normal or abnormal. The abnormal carrier state is defined as the persistent presence of aerobic Gram-negative bacilli (AGNB), including *Klebsiella*, *Enterobacter*, *Proteus*, *Morganella*, *Citrobacter*, *Serratia*,

Acinetobacter and *Pseudomonas* in throat and/or gut [7]. *E. coli* is regarded as a normal microorganism in the gut. During the 1970s two observations on the abnormal carrier state were available: (1) underlying disease promotes persistent abnormal carrying; and (2) antimicrobials that do not respect the gut ecology induce a transient abnormal carrier state in the healthy individual.

In 1969, Johanson showed that disease influences carriage [7]. Varying proportions of patients with such chronic underlying diseases as diabetes, alcoholism, chronic obstructive pulmonary disease (COPD) and liver disease carry abnormal AGNB in the throat and gut. This observation that underlying disease promotes the abnormal carrier state was made independent of antibiotic intake.

Two Dutch groups have demonstrated in healthy animals [8] and in human volunteers [9] that antimicrobials that do not respect the gut ecology may induce transient abnormal carrying, with a return to the normal carrier state two weeks after discontinuation of the antimicrobials that are unfriendly to the indigenous flora. In 1971, van der Waaij quantified the physiological phenomenon of the normal flora controlling the abnormal flora by means of challenge experiments in mice. [8]. He defined colonisation resistance as the concentration of the bacterial challenge strain expressed by the log of colony-forming units per millilitre required to bring about abnormal carriage in half the animals. Generally, healthy animals possess a high colonisation resistance of >9 as they clear high doses of 10^9 AGNB, including *Pseudomonas aeruginosa*, *Klebsiella pneumoniae* and *Enterobacter cloacae*, contaminating their drinking water. Antimicrobials, including cephradine and cefotaxime, do not promote the establishment of abnormal flora and have been labelled ecologically friendly, or "green", antibiotics. The abnormal carrier state was established in 50% of animals that received such antibiotics as ampicillin and flucloxacillin after being challenged with $<10^5$ potentially pathogenic microorganisms (PPM). These agents reduced the resistance of mice to colonisation to <5 and were considered "red" as they disregard the animals gut ecology. Amoxicillin was found to be "amber", as it did not lower the colonisation resistance of mice except when given in high doses.

These antimicrobials were subsequently also tested in healthy volunteers in challenge studies. Vollaard and Clasener demonstrated that none of the antimicrobials were found to be completely ecologically sound [9]. They invariably impacted on colonisation resistance. They argued that the gut flora and fauna is in an extremely fragile balance and highly susceptible to antimicrobial agents. Hence, yeast overgrowth is one of the most common side-effects of antibiotic usage in both 'community' and 'hospital' practice, as one third of individuals are yeast carriers. However, there were still major differences among antimicrobial agents in terms of their influence on the indigenous flora. In the volunteer studies, the effect of ampicillin and amoxicillin on the ecology was significantly worse than that of cephradine and cefotaxime. Abnormal carriage was more frequent and lasted longer with ampicillin and amoxicillin than with cephradine and cefotaxime. The colonisation resistance is mainly based on *Clostridium* species among the indigenous anaerobes. Ampicillin and amoxicillin are intrinsically more potent against *Clostridium* species than cephalosporins. In addition, both antibiotics reach bactericidal concentrations in the faeces following excretion via bile. This combination of factors may explain why the indigenous flora is more affected by ampicillin and amoxicillin than by cephradine and cefotaxime. It has been argued that the effect on colonisation resistance is an important criterion in the selection of antimicrobials.

Setting

The surgical ICU in Groningen became a highly professional organisation with the arrival in 1977 of Professor Dieter Langrehr and Dr Dinis Miranda, who introduced the concept of closed-format ICU organisation according to the Pittsburgh model [10]. "Closed-format" management of an ICU means that the intensivist takes over the management from the previous physician once the patient is admitted to her/his unit. It was an 18-bed unit with four full-time intensivists. Twelve consultants/anaesthetists who were fully trained in intensive care took part in the rota system, at no time were junior doctors in charge of patient care.

Designing Selective Decontamination of the Digestive Tract; a Full Four-Component Strategy: 1979–1986

Surveillance Cultures of Throat and Rectum for Detection of the Abnormal Carrier State

Chris Stoutenbeek was astounded by the high infection rate in the subset of severely traumatized patients who required mechanical ventilation. He met Steven Schimpff, who wrote one of the first papers on infection in trauma patients, which was published in *Annals of Surgery* in 1974 [11]. Following discussions with Steven Schimpff, Chris Stoutenbeek had decided to introduce the use of surveillance samples from throat and rectum in severely traumatised patients [12, 13]. Chris Stoutenbeek reasoned that with the use of diagnostic samples it only would be impossible to unravel the pathogenetic model of infections in this particular subset of critically ill patients requiring ventilation, as surveillance samples from throat and rectum are required to detect the carrier state of a particular micro-organism. Before embarking on a study in trauma patients, he approached Rick van Saene, who had a particular interest, as well as experience, in surveillance cultures in different subsets of immunocompromised populations, including patients with neutropenia and liver transplant recipients [14]. A specialised laboratory in the University Hospital of Groningen, dedicated mainly to monitoring of the level of carriage of potential pathogens by means of quantitative microbiology of surveillance cultures from throat and rectum of immunoparalysed patients, was known as the "Lab van Saene".

Stoutenbeek and van Saene agreed to undertake a thorough literature study, with the aim of clearly defining epidemiological terms before embarking on any study. The results of their literature search of surveillance cultures were an eye-opener for both, as practically all concepts had already been described, albeit with marked variation in the terms, criteria and denominators. Carriage of imported micro-organisms present in the admission flora was distinguished from carriage of acquired microorganisms. Infection episodes can be due to microorganisms present in the patient's throat and/or gut flora, and these infections are termed endogenous infections. In contrast, exogenous infections are due to microorganisms not present in the critically ill patient's own flora but introduced directly into the lower airways, the bloodstream, a wound or the bladder, bypassing the digestive tract [15]. There are two types of endogenous infection: primary endogenous infections are due to microorganisms present in the admission flora, while secondary endogenous infections to microorganisms not imported in the admission flora but acquired later in throat and gut during treatment in the ICU. Stoutenbeek and van Saene were convinced that the denominator of the epidemiological trauma study should be the patient, who may develop one or more episodes of carriage and/or infection, and that the microbiological end-point of the carrier state should be chosen to distinguish imported from acquired microorganisms rather than the criterion of time.

Chris Stoutenbeek, Durk Zandstra, and Rick van Saene designed a prospective study to be conducted over two years (1979–1980) and involving the use of both diagnostic and surveillance samples from severely traumatised patients requiring ventilation for at least five days [14]. Grounds for exclusion were transfer to the ICU because of infectious problems, and recent antimicrobial medication. The main end-point was classification of potential pathogens carried, in particular abnormal AGNB, into imported or acquired, and of infections into exogenous, primary endogenous and secondary endogenous. Before the arrival of Prof. Dieter Langrehr and Dr. Dinis Miranda, microbiology samples were sent to different laboratories, including the Health Protection Agency and the Hospital Epidemiology Department. As part of the new closed format organisation, these two arranged for both diagnostic and surveillance samples to be examined in 'Lab van Saene', for two reasons: (1) the specialised expertise in working with surveillance cultures required for the study; and (2) the requirement for all results, of both cultures and Gram-staining, to be ready before midday. A daily 'micro' meeting was implemented at the ICU from 12:00 noon to –1:00 p.m., with all disciplines involved represented: intensivists, microbiologists, radiologists, surgeons and pharmacists. These daily meetings turned out to be crucial. as they were the forum in which new concepts were conceived and tested. It was at these daily discussions that the four steps in the development of selective digestive tract decontamination (SDD) were established.

Hygiene

Twenty-five years ago, the guidelines recommended by experts and influential institutions included high standards of hygiene and not prescribing and giving antimicrobials until after the infection was diagnosed. The end-point of the five infection control manoeuvres of hand disinfection, isolation, personal protective equipment (gloves, gowns and aprons), care of patient's equipment and environment is control of transmission of potential pathogens via the hands of health-care workers. Transmission of potential pathogens invariably leads to nosocomial, i.e. exogenous and secondary endogenous, infections, and prophylactic antimicrobials are associated with antimicrobial resistance.

The first observational study was undertaken in 59 patients [16–18]. No antibiotic prophylaxis was given. Maintenance of a high level of hygiene was the only prophylactic measure applied, and parenteral antibiotics were not started until an infection was confirmed by microbiological tests. The patients who took part in this baseline study served as the control group later compared with the subsequent three interventions. The infection rate was 81%, with 48 patients developing 94 infection episodes, 35 of which were lower airway infections. It was found that 37% and 28% of the severely traumatised patients were carrying abnormal flora in the oropharyngeal and rectal flora, respectively, on admission. Over the two weeks following admission, these proportions steadily increased to 86% and 76%, respectively. Of the lower airway infections, 75% were primary endogenous, 20% were secondary endogenous and 5% were exogenous. Most of the primary endogenous lower airway infections were due to *Streptococcus pneumoniae*, *Staphylococcus aureus* and *Haemophilus influenzae*, *Pseudomonas aeruginosa*, *Klebsiella*, *Escherichia coli*, *Proteus* and *Enterobacter* species were the causative AGNB of the secondary endogenous lower airway infections. *Acinetobacter* and *Pseudomonas* species caused exogenous lower airway infections. Five (8%) trauma patients died.

Enteral Nonabsorbable Antimicrobials to Convert 'Abnormal' Into 'Normal' Carriage

Rick van Saene prepared a synthesis of the earlier observations and made it clear that the absence of gut contamination with AGNB is due to an individual's good health. Only general well-being guarantees the efficacy of the carriage defence, which is defined as the individual's overall defence mechanism based on seven innate host factors aimed at clearance of AGNB: (1) intact anatomy of mucosal cell lining preventing adherence; (2) physiology, including pH of saliva and stomach; (3) motility maintained by actions of chewing, swallowing and peristalsis; (4) mucosal cell turnover, resulting in sloughing of cells and adherent microorganisms; (5) presence of secretory immunoglobulin A, preventing adherence by coating AGNB; (6) washing effect and stasis prevention by the quality and quantity of secretions such as saliva, bile, gastric fluid, and mucus; and (7) indigenous flora providing colonisation resistance, constituting the microbial factor in carriage defence. The indigenous anaerobic flora is thought to operate in four ways:

- The predominant anaerobes form a "living wallpaper" and occupy the mucosal receptor sites, inhibiting adherence of the incoming abnormal bacteria.

- The anaerobes "starve" the AGNB as they consume huge amounts of nutrients.
- The anaerobic flora produce toxic substances and volatile fatty acids to "knock out" AGNB.
- The anaerobic flora contribute to the clearance of abnormal bacteria via their role in promoting physiological processes, including motility and mucosal cell renewal.

Most importantly, the healthy state implies that there are no receptors on the digestive tract mucosa for adherence of AGNB. A fibronectin layer covering the mucosal cell surface has been hypothesised to protect the host from adhering AGNB. Significantly increased levels of salivary elastase have been shown to precede AGNB carriage in the oropharynx of postoperative patients. It is probable that in individuals suffering both chronic and acute underlying illness, circulating populations of activated macrophages release elastase into mucosal secretions, thereby denuding the protective fibronectin layer. This hypothetical mechanism is thought to be a deleterious consequence of the inflammatory response encountered during and after illness. Currently, the shift of flora from normal to abnormal AGNB in individuals with underlying disease is thought to depend on the severity of the illness. The use of antimicrobials that impair the microbial factor of the carriage defence further promotes gut contamination and overgrowth of abnormal flora. The most profound effects on the patient's ecology and disruption of colonisation resistance have been seen with such extended-spectrum beta-lactam antibiotics as amoxicillin and clavulanic acid, piperacillin and tazobactam, and ceftriaxone. Aminoglycosides have only minor effects on the indigenous gut flora. Fluoroquinolones – while having only limited activity against anaerobes – promote yeast overgrowth. Elimination of faecal AGNB by intravenous ciprofloxacin lowers the rate of molecular oxygen consumption, permitting an increase in the pO_2 of the lumen contents from 5 to 60 mmHg; in such conditions strictly anaerobic microorganisms can no longer survive, even though they may not themselves be sensitive to ciprofloxacin, and yeast overgrowth may subsequently develop owing to an impaired microbial factor in carriage defence. The most logical approach to minimising the risk of PPM overgrowth in the digestive tract is simple, but unfortunately it is not often given much consideration when decisions on antibiotics are made. SDD is based on the concept that the severity of an illness promotes the abnormal carrier state and that drugs including antimicrobials promote overgrowth of abnormal flora.

In 1950, Jacob Fine, a surgeon, described the phenomenon of AGNB leaving the lumen of the gut and migrating into the peritoneal cavity [19]. He termed this process 'transmural migration', as live gut bacteria left the gut through the intestinal mucosal lining and went into the normally sterile peritoneal cavity. Thirty years later Fine's original observation was given the new name 'translocation', defined as the movement of microorganisms from the intestinal lumen to mesenteric lymph nodes, other organs, and blood [20]. Patients with febrile neutropenia develop bloodborne infections following translocation, owing to severe neutropenia ($<100 \times 10^6$ neutrophils/mL [21]. Also in the 1950s, Fine and his colleagues developed the hypothesis that an intestinal endotoxin derived from intraluminal AGNB was the gut-derived toxic factor responsible for the irreversibility in traumatic shock in the presence of sterile blood cultures [22]. The hypothesis was set up that this endotoxin caused fever in severe neutropenia with negative blood cultures. In 1954, Storey, using surveillance cultures, demonstrated that practically all urinary tract infections were preceded by rectal carriage of identical causative AGNB [15].

In 1972, Johanson showed that abnormal oropharyngeal carriage was an independent risk factor for lower airway infections with identical abnormal AGNB [23]. Apart from demonstrating that the oropharynx is the source of bacteria causing pneumonia, Johanson has repeatedly shown that abnormal oropharyngeal carriage develops owing to the severity of an individual's illness, quite independently of antibiotic therapy. Of a series of critically ill patients admitted to a medical intensive care unit 45% developed abnormal carriage: half of these were already abnormal carriers on admission, and the other half became oropharyngeal carriers of AGNB within the first 4 days, which is the period when patients' illness is most severe and the associated immunoparalysis is at its nadir.

Chris Stoutenbeek, Durk Zandstra and Rick van Saene were convinced that the abnormal carrier state harms the patients and that conversion of the 'abnormal' carrier state to the 'normal' carrier state is pivotal in the management of the critically ill patient, as this type of patient is unable to clear abnormal flora owing to the underlying disease [24]. The theoretical foundation on which SDD is based is the concept of 'abnormal carriage' caused by underlying disease and impaired colonisation resistance. An antibiotic protocol was designed to decontaminate (i.e., to eradicate contamination if already present or to prevent it) throat and gut (i.e., the digestive tract) from abnormal bacteria, in particular *P. aeruginosa*, a bacterium associated with ICUs. Anti-pseudomonal antimicrobials, preferably with anti-endotoxin properties, were required; these antibiotics should leave the indigenous, mainly anaerobic, flora largely undisturbed (i.e. be selective) as the normal ecology is thought to contribute to defence against abnormal carriage. It has been proposed that "selectivity" contributes to the "efficacy" of these antibiotics in controlling yeasts [24]. However, there is no evidence that anti-pseudomonal agents that are given parenterally and respect gut flora promote efficacy in clearing abnormal AGNB such as *P. aeruginosa* from throat and gut. The three researchers preferred to rely on high intraluminal levels of lethal antibiotics in saliva and faeces to achieve successful SDD. They searched for a potent anti-pseudomonal combination, using synergistic antimicrobials with low- to moderate-level inactivation by saliva and faeces. They also felt these antimicrobials should be nonabsorbable, to guarantee high intraluminal concentrations.

At the beginning of the 1980s, three decontamination regimens being assessed in neutropenic patients turned out to have some value in eradicating the abnormal carrier state: gentamicin, vancomycin and nystatin (GVN) [25]; framycetin (neomycin), colistin (polymyxin E) and nystatin (FRACON) [26]; and trimethoprim-sulphamethoxazole combined with polymyxin E and amphotericin B (SXTPAM) [27]. However, surveillance cultures invariably showed a high failure rate in attempts to eradicate AGNB, in particular *Pseudomonas aeruginosa*, using these three decontamination protocols. Rick van Saene and Chris Stoutenbeek analysed the surveillance data with the aim of devising an improved decontamination protocol.

They considered an enteral polymyxin essential in any decontamination regimen, for the following reasons. Polymyxins are nonabsorbable and deal with AGNB, including *P. aeruginosa* [28]. However, polymyxins are not active against *Proteus*, *Morganella* and *Serratia* species [29]. Polymyxins are selective in that they are not active against the indigenous, mainly anaerobic, flora. Their mode of action is disruption of the bacterial cell wall, making the bacterial cell permeable and thus readily leading to cell death. This mechanism is independent of enzymatic systems, and acquired resistance to polymyxins is therefore extremely uncommon. Polymyxins are inactivated to a moderate extent by proteins, fibre, food, cell debris, and salivary and faecal compounds and should therefore be given at a relatively high daily dose of 400 mg of polymyxin E (300 mg of polymyxin B) [27]. Polymyxins should be combined with an aminoglycoside owing to the lacking activity against *Proteus*, *Morganella* and *Serratia* species. The aminoglycoside should be active against *P. aeruginosa* because the polymyxins lose activity against this common ICU bacterium in the presence of faeces. Polymyxins neutralise endotoxin. Aminoglycosides have several attractive features for enteral use. They are active against a wide range of AGNB including *P. aeruginosa* and have a potent bactericidal activity similar to that of polymyxins; and there is also synergistic activity with polymyxins [30]. Anti-pseudomonal aminoglycosides include gentamicin, tobramycin and amikacin. They are nonabsorbable and bactericidal, an effect obtained by inhibition of protein synthesis [31]. Tobramycin is the least inactivated by faeces, followed by amikacin and gentamicin [32]. Tobramycin is considered to be selective in terms of leaving the indigenous flora undisturbed at doses lower than 500 mg/day [33]. Low blood concentrations of less than 1 mg/L have been measured [34]. Although the three anti-pseudomonal aminoglycosides and the polymyxins are similar in their bactericidal activity, the total daily dose recommended for tobramycin is 320 mg, lower than the 400 mg for the polymyxins, which are inactivated to a moderate extent by faecal material. The enteral administration of a single aminoglycoside is associated with a substantial failure of decontamination when AGNB – whether sensitive or resistant to gentamicin – are concerned [35]. Aminoglycosides require the addition of polymyxins, as the emergence of aminoglycoside-neutralizing enzymes is not uncommon. Polymyxins are thought to protect tobramycin from being inactivated by faecal enzymes. Tobramycin reduces endotoxin release.

Rick van Saene and Chris Stoutenbeek agreed that an enteral polyene amphotericin B or nystatin was pivotal in any decontamination protocol designed to control yeast overgrowth following the realisation that any antibiotic, whether parenterally or enterally administered, invariably impacts on patient's ecology [9]. Although it is uncommon for oropharyngeal yeast overgrowth to lead to pneumonia following aspiration, gut overgrowth with yeasts had been recognised as an independent risk factor for translocation from the terminal ileum into blood, peritoneum and pancreas causing fungaemia, peritonitis and pancreatitis [36]. Yeast infections of vagina, bladder and skin, including groins and perineum, are invariably preceded by rectal overgrowth [37]. The two polyenes used as decontaminating agents were amphotericin B and nystatin. These are fungicidal and highly selective, as fungi are the only PPM affected by polyenes. They bind to a sterol of the plasma membrane, alter the membrane permeability of the fungal cell leading to the leakage of essential metabolites, and finally fungal cell lysis occurs. Absorption of polyenes is minimal, and the emergence of resistance to polyenes amongst yeasts and fungi is very uncommon. Faecal inactivation of polyenes is high, explaining the high daily doses of 2 g of amphotericin B and of $8x10^6$ units of nystatin that are required for decontamination purposes [38–40].

Enteral vancomycin to eradicate methicillin-sensitive *Staphylococcus aureus* was omitted, as most first-generation cephalosporins clear *S. aureus* from throat and gut [41]. Enteral vancomycin controls methicillin-resistant *S. aureus* (MRSA), but that particular potential pathogen did not cause any problem in trauma patients 25 years ago [42].

Rick van Saene, Chris Stoutenbeek and Durk Zandstra reasoned that the addition of the aminoglycoside neomycin as used in the FRACON protocol or of trimethoprim sulphamethoxazole as part of the SXTPAM regimen to polymyxin did not provide any advantage or improvement over the polymyxin/tobramycin combination, for the following reasons. Neither neomycin nor trimethoprim sulphamethoxazole has anti-pseudomonal or anti-endotoxin activity. In addition, a substantial proportion of patients receiving FRACON and SXTPAM carried AGNB resistant to neomycin and trimethoprim sulphamethoxazole, and *P. aeruginosa*. Although their analysis of surveillance cultures during FRACON and SXTPAM demonstrated suboptimal efficacy in conversion of the abnormal to the normal carrier state, they undertook a pilot study using SXTPAM, as the oncologists at the University Hospital of Groningen claimed to have had positive experience with SXTPAM [27]. This pilot study using SXTPAM was commenced in 1981 in patients staying more than 5 days in the ICU [43]. The oral antibiotic regimen consisted of polymyxin E, 4x200 mg, trimethoprim–sulphamethoxazole, 3x160 mg trimethoprim combined with 800 mg sulphamethoxazole, and amphotericin B, 4x500 mg. Frequent rinsing with chlorhexidine 2% aqueous solution was applied to decontaminate the oropharynx. This regimen of SXTPAM and chlorhexidine rinses was prescribed for 55 patients: 32 multiple trauma patients, 5 cardiac surgery patients and 18 septic patients. Of the 55 patients included in the pilot study, 18 carried abnormal flora in throat and gut, in particular *Pseudomonas* and *Acinetobacter* species. These isolates were sensitive to polymyxin, but resistant to trimethoprim–sulphamethoxazole, confirming observations recorded in previous studies using surveillance cultures. Twelve patients (22%) developed pneumonia. Trimethoprim–sulphamethoxazole is absorbable, but in critically ill patients the absorption is unpredictable, making it necessary to monitor plasma levels in patients with renal impairment. In addition, severe side-effects, including thrombocytopenia and allergy, were observed. Chris Stoutenbeek and Rick van Saene decided to evaluate polymyxin/tobramycin/amphotericin B(PTA), as their negative experience with SXTPAM was in line with their surveillance analysis. Their choice of polymyxin/tobramycin was also supported by the endotoxin research undertaken by Joris van Saene for his PhD [44–46]. The enteral combination of polymyxin/tobramycin had been shown to reduce the faecal endotoxin load significantly, by a factor of 10^4. SDD is based on the concept of the ‘abnormal’ carrier state that is acknowledged to harm the critically ill. The aim of enteral antimicrobials is the control of both primary abnormal (on admission) and secondary (acquired later on during treatment in the ICU) abnormal carriage, in order to prevent endogenous infections. The three investigators at the University of Groningen were the first to evaluate enteral antimicrobials in critically ill patients with multiple trauma [16–18].

Gastrointestinal Eradication of Abnormal Carriage of AGNB Using Enteral Polymyxin/Tobramycin

In a second cohort study, 17 multiple-trauma patients received a 10 ml suspension of polymyxin E 100 mg, tobramycin 80 mg, and amphotericin B 500 mg by nasogastric tube four times daily throughout their treatment in the ICU [18]. No systemic antibiotics were given prophylactically. Ten trauma patients (59%) developed 13 lower airway infections, 10 of which were primary and 3 secondary, endogenous infections. The primary endogenous lower airway infections were invariably due to the normal ‘community’ respiratory pathogens including *S. pneumoniae*, *H. influenzae* and *S. aureus*. *P. aeruginosa* and *A. baumannii* caused the secondary endogenous pneumonias. SDD of stomach and gut did not impact on pneumonia. Two (12%) of the patients died.

Oropharyngeal and Gastrointestinal Eradication of Abnormal Flora Using Enteral Nonabsorbable Antimicrobials

Johanson, who demonstrated in the early 1970s that abnormal oropharyngeal carriage was the major source of lower airway infections with AGNB, was unable to decontaminate the oropharynx. He criticised a positive randomised controlled trial (RCT)[47–49] in which a polymyxin aerosol was used for the prevention of AGNB pneumonia by the Boston group [50]. This well-known Beth Israel RCT was based on the first experience with ventilatory support during the polio epidemic of the 1950s, which demonstrated that topical polymyxin prevented the acquisition of *P. aeruginosa* [29]. Johanson’s two main criticisms were that polymyxin prophylaxis (1) did not prevent death from pneumonia and (b) was associated with the emergence of antimicrobial resistance. Neither of them was valid. There was no acquired resistance in the RCT, but only selection of microorganisms naturally resistant to polymyxins such as *Proteus*,

Serratia and enterococci. Secondly, the Boston RCT was not a mortality study, as the small sample size made it impossible to address that endpoint. In addition, it might be questioned whether enterococcal pneumonia actually kills ICU patients. Subsequently, the Boston investigators were unable to recommend their polymyxin aerosol method for the control of pneumonia. Rick van Saene and Chris Stoutenbeek's choice of polymyxin as the pivotal decontaminating agent was also reinforced for the oropharynx. Tobramycin should be added to polymyxin to control *Proteus* and *Serratia* species. Although polymyxin by aerosol reduced AGNB pneumonia, in particular that attributable to *P. aeruginosa*, the oropharynx was not properly decontaminated in the Boston study. Remarkably, it was Bodey who wrote in 1981 that "antibiotic prophylaxis was less effective against the flora of the throat, probably because of the short contact of antibiotic with the oral mucosa" [51]. Contact time is not guaranteed following sprays, aerosols and mouthwashes, which is in line with the pilot study of SXTPAM [43] and chlorhexidine rinses, which showed a substantial failure rate of oral decontamination of AGNB. The solution came from the experience in dentistry of gels and pastes, which are commonly used precisely because of the prolonged contact time they allow between salivary microorganisms and chlorhexidine and metronidazole mixed with gels and pastes [52, 53]. It was the clinical pharmacist at the University Hospital of Groningen, Marianne Laseur, who prepared a 2% PTA paste at the request of Chris Stoutenbeek [54].

The third step undertaken in the clinical project on antibiotic prophylaxis in multiple trauma patients was the administration of both gut and oropharyngeal SDD, without systemic prophylaxis [18]. Twenty-five trauma patients each received 2 g of a 2% PTA paste applied to the buccal mucosa, combined with 40 ml of a PTA solution into the stomach and gut daily in four doses. The pneumonia rate was 52%, as thirteen patients developed a total of 13 lower airway infections, all of which were due to "community" respiratory pathogens. Although the reduction was not significant, the finding that secondary endogenous pneumonias attributable to abnormal AGNB were completely prevented by oropharyngeal decontamination was striking. One patient (4%) died. For the first time, successful prevention, and eradication if already present, of the abnormal carrier state, both oropharyngeal and intestinal, was achieved. Although Johanson was the first, in 1984, to visit Groningen to congratulate the group of young investigators on their original findings, he never supported SDD [55]. Worse, he even tried to claim SDD as his own original finding in baboons [56].

Immediate Adequate Antimicrobial Therapy to Control Primary Endogenous Infections

It was Jacob Fine who wrote in 1952 that critically ill patients require immediate adequate antimicrobial therapy, which should not be postponed pending microbiology data [57], the main end-point being survival. At the end of the 1960s, bloodborne infections with AGNB, in particular *P. aeruginosa*, involved a high mortality rate in patients with < $100x10^6$ neutrophils/mL [58]. With the advent of carbenicillin and gentamicin, administered immediately in the case of febrile neutropenia, survival improved significantly [59].

Patients who need intensive care because of an acute trauma invariably have invasive devices, including ventilation tube, urinary catheter, and intravascular lines, placed. These interventions are well known risk factors for lower airway, bladder and bloodstream infections in the ICU patient, whose immunoparalysis is at its nadir during the first week after admission. This is the period during which primary endogenous infections occur. Only the immediate administration of parenteral antimicrobials can prevent this type of infection and allow early treatment of an already incubating primary endogenous infection. If the primary endogenous infection is the reason for admission to the ICU, parenteral antimicrobials are required to treat the established infection. Chris Stoutenbeek was convinced that a critically ill patient requiring mechanical ventilation needs immediate administration of parenteral antimicrobials. Hence, parenteral antibiotics are an integral part of the concept of the prophylactic protocol of SDD [60]. Supplementary prophylaxis is the second reason for its use [61]: cover during establishment of SDD on mucosal surfaces, cover for procedurally released microorganisms [62] and elimination of PPM resistant to the enteral antimicrobials from mucosal surfaces; for example, *S. pneumoniae* is resistant to polymyxins, aminoglycosides, and polyenes. Cefotaxime was chosen for the following reasons [63]: (a) its spectrum of activity includes 'normal' respiratory pathogens and 'abnormal' bacteria except for *P. aeruginosa*, *A. baumannii* and MRSA; (b) its pharmacokinetic properties include a high excretion in the target organs, particularly in the bronchial secretions; (c) protein binding is low; and (d) it has a good safety profile.

The fourth observational study undertaken by the Groningen group involved 63 patients admitted to the ICU between 1982 and 1983 [16–18]. They received enteral antimicrobials PTA in throat and gut combined with a parenteral antibiotic, cefotaxime (50–100 mg/kg per day). Cefotaxime was given immediately on admission and was discontinued when PPM were cleared from the oropharynx and the lower airway secretions were sterile. Five trauma patients (8%) developed lower airway infections with an exogenous pathogenesis; as primary endogenous lower airway infections disappeared and there were no secondary endogenous infections attributable to the enteral antibiotics. There were no deaths in this subset of patients who received both parenteral and enteral antimicrobials.

By 1983 the new concept of antimicrobial prophylaxis using four components in ICU patients had taken shape. There was a new method by which the abnormal carrier state could be converted into normal carriage using enteral agents. The internal organs, including lower airways and blood, could be kept sterile following immediate administration of adequate parenteral antimicrobials. High standards of hygiene and regular surveillance cultures together with the parenteral and enteral antimicrobials are the four components of SDD. Thus, the Stoutenbeek tetralogy was born, and subsequently the first RCT assessing SDD in trauma patients was undertaken in Groningen from 1984 to 1986 [64].

The publication of the first observational results [16–18] generated a great deal of interest, and well-known researchers came to Groningen to learn about the new method with the intention of starting clinical trials themselves. Professor Ledingham, of Glasgow (Scotland), was amongst the first, followed by several German investigators, including G. Hünefeld (Hanover), F. Konrad (Ulm), M. Sydow (Göttingen) and U. Hartenauer (Münster). Ruud Krom introduced SDD into the USA following his appointment as liver transplant surgeon at the Mayo Clinics in Rochester [65].

Van der Waaij and Sluiter, professors of Medical Microbiology and Respiratory Medicine, respectively, opposed SDD in the critically ill patient. They adopted this position mainly because of the unpleasant taste of polymyxin and because of the choice of tobramycin, which was thought to disturb patients' colonisation resistance to a greater degree than aztreonam and temocillin [66–68]. Since hard scientific evidence against the new approach was lacking, the capital sin of the group of young researchers lay in failing to comply with expert expectations in the use of antibiotic prophylaxis. The three investigators were invited by Professor Ledingham to write a chapter on the concepts and results of SDD. Political manoeuvres, including intimidation, resulted in a chapter entitled, 'The control of Gram-negative bacterial infection in the ICU' with Prof. Dieter Langrehr and Dr Dinis Miranda as the only two authors and Professor van der Waaij's contribution acknowledged as "careful reading of the manuscript" [69]. The Chief Executive, Mr Hamel supported the surgeons, and Professor Langrehr took early retirement. This climate of intrigue was not unfamiliar in Groningen [70] and inhibited further clinical research there; in 1987, Chris Stoutenbeek and Durk Zandstra left for Amsterdam, and Rick van Saene for Liverpool.

Chris Stoutenbeek and Durk Zandstra were appointed as consultant/intensive medicine specialists in an 18-bedded intensive care unit for medical/surgical adult patients at the Onze-Lieve-Vrouwe-Gasthuis in Amsterdam. Chris Stoutenbeek was called to the Chair of Intensive Care Medicine at the University of Amsterdam seven years later, in 1994. Neither surveillance cultures to detect the abnormal carrier state nor selective decontamination were in use in the adult units the two had gone to from Groningen. However, traditional surveillance of infection was in place, which revealed a serious problem with pneumonia and septicaemia. Tragically, Chris Stoutenbeek was diagnosed with end-stage non-Hodgkin lymphoma in the summer of 1997. Chemotherapy and bone marrow transplantation failed, and Chris Stoutenbeek died of post-transplant lymphoproliferative disease in 1999.

Rick van Saene was appointed as senior lecturer in Medical Microbiology at the University of Liverpool (U.K.) and honorary consultant microbiologist at the Royal Liverpool Children's Hospital of Alder Hey. In spite of a tough resistance to process surveillance cultures among the BMS staff, he transformed a traditional department processing diagnostic samples only into one providing a laboratory service based on both surveillance and diagnostic samples. The abnormal carrier state was indicative for the commencement of SDD. Unlike other units, in which SDD is started on admission, Alder Hey uses knowledge of the carrier state as a marker. This experience has recently been published in *Critical Care Medicine* by the intensivist Dr Richard Sarginson. That publication was based on the largest SDD database, including results of both diagnostic and surveillance samples. Nia Taylor, a database expert, joined the SDD team at Alder Hey in 1999. The vast amount of data is entered into the database, which is unique in that it not only surveys infection, but also the carrier state over 8 years. All patients who are carriers of MRSA and/or ceftazidime-/tobramycin-resistant AGNB are registered, in addition to patients infected with the resistant bacteria mentioned above. Knowledge of the carrier state is required for classification of the infections encountered into exogenous, and primary and secondary endogenous groups. In addition, both enteral (SDD) and parenteral antibiotic usage are recorded.

Twenty years of clinical research on SDD yielded 74 trials, including 46 RCTs [71–126] and 18 non-randomised trials [17, 127–143] and 13 meta-analyses [144–156], three of which included nonrandomised studies [154–156].

Selective decontamination of the digestive tract: the best ever evaluated manoeuvre in ICUs: 1987–2007

Forty-six randomised controlled trials (RCT; Table 1.1)

The first RCT was published in 1987 and originated from Munich, Germany [121]. Professors Gottard Ruckdeschel and Klaus Unertl were the driving forces

Table 1.1. Forty-six randomised controlled trials from Europe

The Netherlands (n = 11)	Utrecht [96], Groningen [117, 126], Amsterdam [95, 118] Rotterdam [101, 119], Maastricht [75], Leiden [79], The Hague [120], Nijmegen [72]
Spain (n = 9)	Murcia [102, 103, 110], Madrid [81, 113, 114], Barcelona [85, 104], La Coruna [109]
United Kingdom (n = 8)	Belfast [77], London [111, 112], Birmingham [76], Nottingham [86], Liverpool [91], Cardiff [94], Bristol [124]
France (n = 7)	Paris [80, 97], Lyon [89], Limoges [88], Rennes [82], Toulouse [90], Marseille [107]
Germany (n = 5)	Munich [71, 98, 115, 121], Berlin [108]
Austria (n = 3)	Vienna [99], Innsbruck [100], Graz [125]
Switzerland (n = 1)	Geneva [106]
Belgium (n = 1)	Leuven [122]
Greece (n = 1)	Athens [105]

in the Munich group, which subsequently published three more RCTs [71, 98, 115]. An RCT in liver transplant recipients was undertaken in Berlin [108]. Professor Daschner, one of the original SDD bashers, has written repeatedly since 1987 that SDD promotes resistance; he still continues in this vein today [157]. During the mid-1980s he swore "SDD mit allen Mitteln nieder zu machen" [to take SDD down in any way I can]. Despite Professor Daschner's opinion, i.e., that only the lowest level of evidence is available, the first individual RCT demonstrating a significant survival benefit in patients receiving SDD was published by the group around Professors Gottard Ruckdeschel and Klaus Unertl in 2002 [98].

The second RCT [96] was published in the following year 1988, and was undertaken in Utrecht, The Netherlands. Dr Hans Rommes initiated, designed and supervised the first Dutch RCT and has been a loyal SDD activist from its inception up to the present [158]. When Dr Hans Rommes moved from Groningen to Utrecht, one of the first things he did was to introduce surveillance cultures to unravel the pathogenesis of infections in surgical ICU patients before embarking on the first Dutch SDD RCT [96, 159]. Ten more trials followed, making The Netherlands the country with the highest number of RCTs on SDD (Table 1.1). While already seriously ill, Chris Stoutenbeek initiated and designed the largest individual trial of SDD in about 1,000 patients, demonstrating an overall reduction of mortality by 8% [95]. However, criticism persisted over the years [160–162].

The first Spanish RCT [110] from Murcia was published in 1990 by A. Martinez. This RCT assessed oropharyngeal decontamination only, without the intestinal and parenteral component, which was never evaluated by the original investigators. The same group published two more RCTs [102, 103] on the role of SDD in the control of endotoxaemia following cardiovascular bypass surgery. A total of nine Spanish RCTs have been published (Table 1.1). All but one showed a significant reduction in infectious morbidity, including endotoxaemia, following heart surgery. However, Miguel-Angel de la Cal, from Madrid, is currently the most prominent SDD figure in Spain and South America. Miguel-Angel de la Cal is the lead intensivist of the ICU at Getafe, where he launched a comprehensive surveillance programme in both medical/surgical and burns ICUs in 1995 [163]. He is an outstanding clinician and clinical epidemiologist, in addition to being Editor-in-Chief of *Medicina Intensiva*. He initiated and designed the only RCT in burn patients, demonstrating a decline in mortality from 27.8% to 9.4% in patients receiving SDD [81]. He also eradicated MRSA from his ICU [164] and Burns Unit [165].

The first RCT [77] from the United Kingdom was published in 1991 by the group of Lowry in Belfast (Northern Ireland). This RCT was the first with a large sample size (N=331). Of the eight UK trials, three were undertaken in liver transplant recipients [76, 111, 112], two by Prof. Roger Williams in London [111, 112] and one by Julian Bion in Birmingham [76]. The Bristol trial [124] demonstrated a significant reduction in the number of patients with sepsis syndrome following SDD. Since its inception, SDD has rarely received a favourable press, amongst either intensivists [166, 167] or microbiologists in the UK [168, 169].

The first French RCT [80] from Paris, published in 1989, showed the efficacy of SDD as a manoeuvre to control an outbreak caused by expanded spectrum beta-lactamase producing *Klebsiella*. France has produced a total of seven RCTs (Table 1.1). Despite a powerful Parisian anti-SDD movement,[170, 171], the research group in Marseille under the leadership of Claude Martin has persistently applied SDD in trauma–patients [172].

Three RCTs originate from Austria [99, 100, 125] (Table 1.1). Only the RCT conducted in a paediatric cardiac ICU [125] showed a significant reduction in infectious morbidity, whilst those conducted in a mixed ICU [99] and in a trauma RCT in 357 patients [125] gave negative results.

Switzerland, Belgium and Greece have each undertaken one RCT on SDD. The Belgian RCT conducted in a large sample of 600 medical/surgical patients [122] is almost certainly the most misleading of all the 56 RCTs. There was no significant increase in antimicrobial resistance following SDD when the patient was used as the denominator. Therefore, the researchers in Leuven, Belgium, analysed their data by number of isolates, confirming their pre-trial bias toward the view that SDD creates antimicrobial resistance.

There is only one RCT from South Africa, which was undertaken in a respiratory unit [92]. SDD was employed to control endemicity of a multi-resistant *Acinetobacter baumannii*. The reduction in infection was not significant.

Of the fifty-six RCTs, nine (<20%) were undertaken in the USA [73, 74, 78, 83, 84, 87, 93, 116, 123], Bob Weinstein and his group in Chicago were the first, in 1990, to publish their positive RCT in cardiac adult patients [87]. Five years later the same group assessed SDD in a mixed population, with no impact on infection rates [123]. The third trial [73] from Chicago was undertaken in liver transplant recipients. The Mayo Clinics evaluated SDD in a medical/surgical ICU [84] and in liver transplant recipients [93]. The other four US trials originated from Charleston (trauma patients) [78], Pittsburgh (paediatric liver transplant recipients) [116], Minneapolis (surgical ICU) [83] and Galveston (paediatric burns ICU) [74]. Many of the opinion leaders in the USA prefer to criticise the available evidence [173–176].

The six negative RCTs [85, 88, 92, 100, 122, 123] have a few denominators in common: (1) each is published in a journal with a high impact factor; (2) MRSA was endemic in the unit concerned during the RCT; (3) the denominator of infectious morbidity was infection episodes and not number of infected patients; and (4) there was an exogenous problem. During the early 1980s, MRSA was not the problem it is today, so that SDD was designed to reduce pneumonia and septicaemia attributable to AGNB and yeasts. The pathogenesis of acquisition and carriage of and infection with MRSA is identical to that of AGNB and yeasts, the main risk factors being hygiene, severe illness and gut carriage, respectively [177]. Enteral vancomycin applied in the same manner as classic SDD has been shown to prevent carriage of and subsequent infection with MRSA [178].

Ten meta-analyses of only individual trials [144–153]
Half of these were undertaken by Italian researchers, three from the Mario Negro Institute in Milan by the group of A. Liberati [144, 147, 150] and two by L. Silvestri, Head of Department of Intensive Care, Gorizia, Italy [152, 153]. The other five originated from North America. Canadian researchers published two meta-analyses, one performed by the evidence-based medical unit of Prof. David Sackett in Hamilton [145] and one by the Department of Academic Surgery headed by John Marshall in Toronto [148]. Kollef's group published two systematic reviews [146, 149], and Safdar, in Wisconsin, undertook one [151] meta-analysis. Most meta-analyses assessed pneumonia as the morbidity end-point. Bloodstream infection was evaluated in three meta-analyses [148, 149, 153]. All meta-analyses without exception revealed a significant reduction in infectious morbidity. Of the seven meta-analyses with the end-point of mortality, a survival benefit was found in five [144, 145, 147, 148, 150].

Eighteen nonrandomised SDD trials [17, 127–143]
There are five German [128, 129, 131, 133, 139], three English [134–136] and three Dutch [17, 137, 143] nonrandomised studies. Two nonrandomised studies originate from South Africa [138, 140]. Scotland [127], France [132], Italy [130], Australia [141] and Spain [142] have each produced one controlled SDD trial with a nonrandomised design, all of which have been historically controlled.

The first study evaluating enteral and parenteral antimicrobials in trauma patients [17] was the original one published by Chris Stoutenbeek's group in 1984. This first SDD study – albeit nonrandomised – had a major impact on the intensive care community. Stoutenbeek's original observation ranks 19 in the top citation classics in critical care journals [179].

The Scottish study from the Western Infirmary in Glasgow was published by Ian McA. Ledingham in *The Lancet* in 1988 [127]. Ledingham's study promoted the eight RCTs in the United Kingdom and was the stimulus for the three South African trials. In addition, the pharmacy department at the Western Infirmary initiated production of the enteral SDD products. Unfortunately, Ian McA. Ledingham left Glasgow in 1990, leaving behind him a legacy and tradition of SDD that is still as strong today under the guidance of the microbiologist Dr Steve Alcock and the pharmacist Mr K. Pollock.

Three meta-analyses of SDD trials including nonrandomised trials [154–156]
The first ever meta-analysis of SDD-trials was performed in Utrecht, The Netherlands [154]. It was published in 1991 and included eleven studies, five of which were not randomised. Although the Australian meta-analysis of forty studies [155] published in 1995 differentiates between RCTs and non-RCTs, the nonrandomised Hünefeld study was included in the subset of RCTs. The other Dutch meta-analysis [156] published in 2001 from Maastricht, included thirthy-two trials, five of which were not randomised [180]. Surprisingly, Professor Bonten, who supervised the Maastricht meta-analysis, categorises his meta-analysis as one dealing exclusively with prospective randomised trials [181, 182].

All three led to reports of significantly reduced infectious morbidity. Bonten reports an inverse relationship between the quality of study design and the reported effects on pneumonia prevention: with increasingly better study quality the preventive effects became less pronounced, although reductions remained statistically significant even for the best studies. Study quality did not, however, influence the reported reductions in ICU mortality. All but one (Utrecht) of the meta-analyses demonstrate significant survival benefit following SDD.

Six conferences dedicated to SDD [14, 16, 183–186]

Professor Camus from the Free University of Brussels organised a meeting in Brussels in April 1983 with the major aim of presenting the preliminary data on the four steps in the development of SDD [14, 16]. All lectures were subsequently published in the *Acta Anaesthesiologica Belgica* with the end-point of claim of first authorship [14, 16].

Five years later, in 1988, Rick van Saene, Chris Stoutenbeek, Prof. Peter Lawin and Prof. Ian McLedingham organised an international congress on the island of Jersey to compare data obtained with SDD with the results yielded by the conventional approach. The proceedings of this SDD congress were published as a separate volume (no.7) of *Update in Intensive Care and Emergency Medicine* (edited by J.L. Vincent) entitled '*Infection Control by Selective Decontamination*' [183]. This congress constituted the major impetus for the first wave of 25 SDD RCTs in the first half of the 1990s (Figure 1.1).

The European Society for Intensive Care Medicine, in which the French opinion leaders have a major influence, has never been supportive of SDD. Indeed, in November 1991 Prof. Jean Carlet organised the first European Consensus Conference in Paris, France, on 'Selective Decontamination of the Digestive Tract'. Although all participants agreed that the meeting was really successful and stimulat-

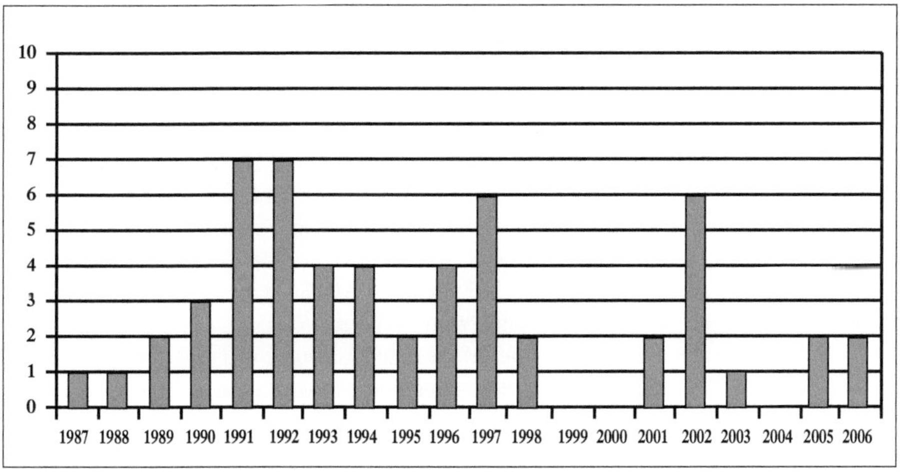

Fig. 1.1 Forty-six randomised trials of SDD from 1987 to 2007

ing, the report was at odds with their experience [184] and set the scene by coming down against SDD; this is in line with the maxim of Prof. David Sackett, the pope of evidence-based medicine: "Consensus does not make sense" [187]. Amazingly, exactly 2 months after the negative Consensus Conference, the French Working Group on SDD published the first negative SDD RCT in the *New England Journal of Medicine* [88]. The conclusion confirmed that of the Consensus report: "SDD does not improve survival, although it substantially increases the cost of ... care." Fortunately, Alessandro Liberati, from the Cochrane Collaboration in Milan, Italy, made an unexpected positive contribution to the Consensus Conference with the first results of the meta-analysis to be published in the BMJ in 1993 [144]. His compatriot, Luciano Silvestri, attended the Consensus Conference in Paris and was excited about the new philosophy. Back in Trieste, he initiated a major clinical research programme based on surveillance cultures, turning Trieste's hospital into the SDD research unit in Italy. Luciano Silvestri is industrious and self-disciplined. His attitude towards completing projects both personal and professional is tenacious. These qualities ensure his position as one of the best clinical researches in ICU-medicine.

Professor Antonino Gullo organised a course of infection control by SDD at the annual APICE meeting 1994. The complete course was published as the first edition of '*Infection Control in ICU*' in the series '*Topics in Anaesthesia and Critical Care*' (edited by A. Gullo) in 1998 [185]. In 2002, at the 17th APICE meeting, a completely updated course on the management of infection in the critically ill using SDD was organised by Professor Gullo. The second edition of '*Infection Control in ICU*' appeared in print in 2005 [186].

In 2002, Peter van der Voort organised a symposium on SDD in Papendal (The Netherlands) under the auspices of the Dutch Society of Intensive Care.

Twenty-one theses on SDD [188–209]
SDD has been the subject of at least 21 thesis studies.

Emergence of a Powerful Anti-SDD Movement

The original opposition was uniquely French. Two experts, Professors Brun-Buisson and Carlet, focused their resistance to SDD on the discrepancy between the 65% reduction in pneumonia by SDD resulting in only a 20% reduction in mortality. They asserted that the absence of a strong correlation between prevention of pneumonia and survival benefit was due to a low specificity for diagnosing pneumonia. Diagnosing pneumonia is difficult, and reported pneumonia rates may have been too high in the absence of SDD because nonspecific diagnostic criteria, e.g., tracheal aspirate, were applied [210] or too low in patients receiving SDD because of leakage of oral antibiotics into the trachea [211]. Over the last 10 years, Kollef and Bonten have profiled themselves as opponents of SDD [176, 212]. Bonten does conduct research into SDD, but so far only partially, as in the first Spanish study from Murcia on oropharyngeal decontamination in 1990. Bonten believes that ICU mortality can be reduced by the topical application of an oropharyngeal antimicrobial gel alone, without the emergence of antimicrobial resistance [75, 213]. In their criticism of SDD some opponents assert that enterococcal pneumonia is a serious side-effect of SDD [214]. However, enterococcal infection can occur during SDD treatment but lead to a relatively low inflammatory state, when it is easy to treat and does not lead to attributable mortality (Table 1.2).

Why is SDD not widely used?

Table 1.2 Statements by experts according to country of origin

Expert, country, year of statement	[Ref.]	Publication data
1. PJ Sanderson, UK, 1989	[168]	BMJ 1989
'The contribution of the parenteral component is not clear and its danger the greatest'		
2. J Carlet, France, 1991	[170]	Lettre 1991
'La DDS, une technique n'ayant fait la preuve ni de son efficacité ni de son innocuité'		
3. A Gilston, UK, 1991	[166]	Intensive Crit Care Dig 1991
'Future candidates for the scrap heap include SDD. …'		
4. DJ Bihari, UK, 1993	[167]	BMJ, 1993
'Until there is good evidence that SDD is beneficial attention to accepted standards are likely to reap greater rewards'		
5. C Brun-Buisson, France, 1993	[171]	Proceedings, Brussels Meeting, 1993
'It is now clear that SDD in all unselected patients is a poorly effective exercise, wasteful of resources and potentially harmful'		
6. J Verhoef, The Netherlands, 1993	[161]	CID 1993
'SDD led to the emergence of resistant micro-organisms'		
7. M Barza, USA, 1993	[173]	AAC 1993
'Routine clinical use of this practice should be discouraged'		
8. JL Vincent, Belgium, 1995		Personal communication
'How can SDD work, when no one's using it?'		
9. R van Furth, The Netherlands, 1995	[160]	Medical Year, 1995
'Well designed research in the Netherlands and elsewhere has demonstrated that SDD on ICU does not improve morbidity and mortality in this subset of patients, and should be stopped'		
10. WM Zapol, USA, 1996	[174]	Br J Anaesth, 1996
'Aspiration of contaminated gastric contents is the main endogenous pathway for lower airway infections. Sucralfate does prevent lower airway infections due to its control of gastric overgrowth, whilst SDD does not work because mortality has never been impacted by that intervention'		

Continue ⟶

Continue **Table 1.2**

Expert, year of statement	[Ref.]	Publication data
11. CG Mayhall, USA, 1997	[175]	Infect Dis Clin N Am, 1997
'The efficacy of SDD for the prevention of nosocomial pneumonia is unproven.'		
12. JL Vincent, Belgium 1999	[214]	Thorax, 1999
'SDD has been based on the hypothesis of colonization resistance'		
13. M Kollef, USA, 1999	[176]	N Engl J Med, 1999
'SDD has not gained acceptance in the US, because of its lack of demonstrated effect on mortality, the emergence of antibiotic-resistant infections, and additional toxicity'		
14. F Daschner, Germany, 2000	[157]	Eur J Clin Microbiol, 2000
'There is no doubt that the use of SDD favours the emergence of bacterial resistance equally among G^+ and G- pathogens.'		
15. CH Webb, UK, 2000	[169]	J Hosp Infect, 2000
'Until its microbiological safety is unequivocally demonstrated, its unselective use is not yet justified'		
16. MJM Bonten, The Netherlands, 2001	[212]	NTvG, 2001
'No SDD for IC patients'		

Two recent reviews of the usage of SDD reveal that it is routinely used in only 4% of UK ICUs [215], but in 24% of Dutch ICUs [216]. The most common reason cited for not using it [83%] is the belief held by UK intensivists that evidence of efficacy is lacking and 'it does not work' [212]. The reason for this misconception is multifactorial. However, the longstanding disagreement amongst experts [214, 218] has been an important factor contributing to the confusion. History repeats itself: Semmelweis' work was heavily opposed by Virchow, the expert pathologist of that time [219].

The main reason why SDD is not widely used is the primacy of opinion over evidence. Previous experience with thrombolytic drugs indicates a similar pattern, with an undesirable lag between the appearance of meta-analytic evidence and the recommendations of experts. Streptokinase was shown to reduce the risk of death from myocardial infarction by 20% as long ago as 1975. During the next two decades 14 review articles either failed to mention streptokinase or referred to it as still experimental [220], although in this century the administration of streptokinase is virtually routine in patients with myocardial infarction.

Concerns expressed about resistance have also hindered the implementation of SDD. All analyses of antimicrobial resistance associated with SDD are based on case reports [157] and review articles [212] rather than on evidence. A statement based on expert opinion is misleading and runs contrary to the aims of EBM: the best estimate based on an impartial review of all available information. One concern is that in many reviews isolates, samples or infections, and not patients, are used as the denominator [122]. All reviews include the seven RCTs which were conducted in ICUs where MRSA was endemic at the time of the trial, although there was only a trend towards a higher MRSA infection rate in the patients receiving SDD [81, 85, 88, 92, 100, 122, 123]. A statistically significant trend towards resistance amongst Gram-positive bacteria was found only after the inclusion of rates of carriage and infection attributable to low-level pathogens such as enterococci and coagulase-negative staphylococci. Clearly, pneumonia due to these low-level pathogens is extremely rare. Finally, exogenous infections are not controlled by SDD. A transient increase in exogenous lower airway infections due to *Acinetobacter baumannii* was reported from a respiratory unit with a high percentage of tracheotomised patients during the course of an RCT on SDD [92]. This observation that the proportion of exogenous infections in SDD trials increases in relation to the reduction in endogenous infections is well recognised. This transient finding is repeatedly used to show that SDD increases resistance amongst AGNB [221]. The assertion that resistance is a problem with SDD is misplaced in an evidence-based analysis.

Since its inception, SDD has rarely received favourable press. A higher acceptance rate for papers recording negative results for SDD compounds its poor reputation – of the fifty-six randomised trials of SDD, the six showing no benefit [85, 88, 92, 100, 122, 123] were all published in journals with high impact factors. An extreme example is the publication in the *New England Journal of Medicine* of an uncontrolled study in which 10% of the study population developed enterococcal pneumonia [216]. It might be questioned whether such a high incidence of such an obscure condition should be taken at face value.

Selective decontamination of the digestive tract has also never been promoted by pharmaceutical companies, perhaps because there is little profit in older agents, such as cefotaxime, polymyxin E, tobramycin and amphotericin B, which are inexpensive and already out of patent. Furthermore, SDD is not supported by authoritative-looking data sheets and is not marketed to clinicians in the traditional manner. Paste, gel and suspension are not readily available on the shelf. Hence, the application of SDD requires more effort from the ICU team in terms of commitment and monitoring than is needed for systemic administration of the latest antibiotic on the market.

Finally, Wazana questions the interaction of physicians and the pharmaceutical industry and asks 'Is a gift ever just a gift?' [222]. Most opinion leaders have links with the industry and receive grants for the evaluation of new antimicrobial agents both in vitro and in vivo. The same experts attend national and international meetings, which they chair and where they report data often promoting these new drugs as first-line antibiotics. The traditionalists on the 'circuit' have relied on the industry to develop new drugs at regular intervals, usually two years following publication of the first case report of superinfections of the currently favoured antibiotic. The realisation that the pharmaceutical industry had failed to provide new classes of antibiotics came as a heavy blow. Industrialised countries have largely delegated control of drug trials to pharmaceutical companies, which places clear limitations on research [223]. However, economic interests seek the best possible financial return, and establishing new and potent antibiotics to treat rather than prevent pneumonia is more profitable. Antibiotic usage in the (UK) National Health Service is determined mainly by the pharmaceutical industry. The replacement of piperacillin by piperacillin/tazobactam illustrates the much greater importance attached to market forces and financial incentives than to public health needs.

The Future: SDD Controls Resistance

Perhaps the most intriguing aspect of the 20 years of clinical research into SDD is the experience that the addition of enteral antibiotics to parenteral antimicrobials may prolong the antibiotic era [224, 225]. Practically all patients who require intensive care for minimally three days have gut overgrowth defined as $\geq 10^5$ AGNB per gram of faeces, owing to increased gastric pH of >4 and impaired peristalsis [226]. Gut overgrowth guarantees increased spontaneous mutation, associated with polyclonality and antimicrobial resistance. Enteral polymyxin and tobramycin eradicate carriage, overgrowth and resistant mutants, preventing the emergence of antimicrobial resistance [224]. Pre-1980 antibiotics are still active so long as they are combined with eradication of aerobic gram-negative bacilli and MRSA from the gut. We believe that the answer lies not in the development of single, new, more potent and expensive systemic antimicrobials, but in a radical re-think of the philosophy according to which antimicrobials are used. In particular, we need to be much more critical of market-driven health care if we are to find more sustainable solutions to the problems of the ongoing spread of nosocomial, antibiotic-resistant pathogens in the new millennium.

In spite of the powerful anti-SDD movement, SDD is now an EBM protocol. Influential European, UK and US societies and institutions acknowledge that SDD is the best-ever evaluated intervention in intensive care medicine that reduces infectious morbidity and mortality [227–230]. The US Department for Health and Human Services considers SDD to be a cheap manoeuvre [230].

The current project is the SDD website, www.SDD.web.com, of which Miss Norma Aspinall is in charge. The website will contain everything you need to know about SDD, including a complete literature database, practical guidelines and procurement information. There will be a forum for questions and answers and a discussion board. We hope to have the site up and running early in 2007, and it is our intention to update it regularly.

A follow-up to the Jersey meeting is planned for 2008, when 20 years of clinical SDD research and developments will be evaluated.

The third project is the third edition of '*Infection Control in ICU*' to be published in 2012.

References

1. Feingold DS (1970) Hospital-acquired infections. N Engl J Med 283:1384-1391
2. Eickhoff TC, Brachmann PS, Bennett JV et al (1969) Surveillance of nosocomial infections in community hospitals. I. Surveillance methods, effectiveness and initial results. J Infect Dis 120:305-317
3. Daschner FD, Frey P, Wolff G et al (1982) Nosocomial infections in intensive care wards : a multi-centre prospective study. Intensive Care Med 8:5-9
4. Northey D, Adess ML, Hartsuck JM et al (1974) Microbiological surveillance in surgical intensive care unit. Surg Gynecol Obstet 139:321-325
5. Fry DE, Pearlstein L, Fulton RL et al (1980) Multiple organ system failure (the role of uncontrolled infection). Arch Surg 115:136-140
6. Goris RJA, Draaisma J (1982) Causes of death after blunt trauma. J Trauma 22:141-146
7. Johanson WG, Pierce AK, Sanford JP (1969) Changing pharyngeal bacterial flora of hospitalised patients. Emergence of Gram-negative bacilli. N Engl J Med 281:1137-1140
8. van der Waaij D (1992) History of recognition and measurement of colonization resistance of the digestive tract as an introduction to selective gastro-intestinal decontamination. Epidemiol Infect 109:315-326
9. Vollaard EJ, Clasener HAL (1994) Colonization resistance. Antimicrob Agents Chemother 335:409-414
10. Safar P, Grenvik A (1977) Organisation and physician education in critical care medicine. Anaesthesiology 47:82-95
11. Schimpff SC, Miller RM, Polakavetz S et al (1974) Infection in the severely traumatized patient. Ann Surg 179:352-357
12. Schimpff SC (1981) Surveillance cultures. J Infect Dis 144:81-84
13. Schimpff SC, Young VM, Greene WH et al (1972) Origin of infection in acute non-lymphocytic leukaemia. Significance of hospital acquisition of potential pathogens. Ann Intern Med 77:707-714
14. van Saene HKF, Stoutenbeek CP, Miranda DR et al (1983) A novel approach to infection control in the intensive care unit. Acta Anaesth Belg 34:193-209
15. Storey P (1954) Proteus infections in hospital. J Pathol Bacteriol 68:55-62
16. Stoutenbeek CP, van Saene HKF, Miranda DR et al (1983) A new technique of infection prevention in the intensive care unit by selective decontamination of the digestive tract. Acta Anaesth Belg 34:209-221
17. Stoutenbeek CP, van Saene HKF, Miranda DR et al (1984) The effect of selective decontamination of the digestive tract on colonization and infection rate in multiple trauma patients. Intensive Care Med 10:185-192
18. Stoutenbeek CP, van Saene HKF, Miranda DR et al (1987) The effect of oropharyngeal decontamination using topical non-absorbable antibiotics on the incidence of nosocomial respiratory tract infections in multiple trauma patients. J Trauma 27:357-364
19. Schweinburg FB, Seligman AM, Fine J (1950) Transmural migration of intestinal bacteria. N Engl J Med 242:747-751
20. Berg RD, Garlington AW (1979) Translocation of certain indigenous bacteria from the gastrointestinal tract to the mesenteric lymph nodes and other organs in a gnotobiotic mouse model. Infect Immun 23:403-411
21. Bodey GP, Buckley M, Sathe YS et al (1966) Quantitative relationships between circulating leucocytes and infection in patients with acute leukaemia. Ann Intern Med 64:328-340
22. Fine J, Frank ED, Rutenberg SH et al (1959) The bacterial factor in traumatic shock. N Engl J Med 260:214-216
23. Johanson WG, Pierce AK, Sanford JP et al (1972) Nosocomial respiratory tract infections with Gram-negative bacilli. The significance of colonization of the respiratory tract. Ann Intern Med 77:701-706
24. van Saene HKF, Stoutenbeek CP (1987) Selective decontamination. J Antimicrob Chemother 20:462-465

25. Levine AS, Siegel SE, Schreiber AD et al (1973) Protected environments and prophylactic antibiotics. A prospective controlled study of their utility in the therapy of acute leukaemia. N Engl J Med 288:477-483
26. Storring RA, Jameson B, McElwain TJ et al (1977) Oral non-absorbed antibiotics prevent infection in acute non-lymphoblastic leukaemia. Lancet II:837-840
27. Kurrle E, Dekker AW, Gaus W et al (1986) Prevention of infection in acute leukaemia: A prospective randomised study on the efficacy of two different drug regimens for antimicrobial prophylaxis. Infection 14:226-232
28. Hoeprich PD (1970) The polymyxins. Med Clin North Am 54:1257-1265
29. Lepper MH, Kofman S, Blatt N et al (1954) Effect of eight antibiotics used simply and in combination on the tracheal flora following tracheotomy in poliomyelitis. Antibiot Chemother 4:829-843
30. Kuipers JS (1975) Combinations of antimicrobial agents. I. The in vitro sensitivity of 100 strains of Pseudomonas aeruginosa to polymyxin B, colistin, carbenicillin, gentamicin and doxycycline and to various combinations of these antibiotics. Arch Chir Neerl 27:257-270
31. Neu HC (1976) Tobramycin: an overview. J Infect Dis 134:S3-S19
32. van Saene JJM, van Saene HKF, Stoutenbeek CP et al (1985) Influence of faeces on the activity of antimicrobial agents used for decontamination of the alimentary canal. Scand J Infect Dis 17:295-300
33. Mulder JG, Wiersma WE, Welling GW et al (1984) Low dose oral tobramycin treatment for selective decontamination of the digestive tract: a study in human volunteers. J Antimicrob Chemother 13:495-504
34. Bodey GP, Pan T (1980) Absorption of tobramycin after chronic oral administration. Curr Ther Res 28:394-401
35. Klastersky J, DeBusscher L, Weerts D et al (1974) Use of oral antibiotics in protected units environment: clinical effectiveness and role in the emergence of antibiotic-resistant strains. Pathol Biol 22:5-12
36. van Saene HKF, Damjanovic V, Pizer B et al (1999) Fungal infections in ICU. J Hosp Infect 41:337-340
37. Miles MR, Olsen L, Rogers A (1977) Recurrent vaginal candiasis. Importance of an intestinal reservoir. JAMA 238:1836-1837
38. Bodey GP (1969) The effect of amphotericin B on the fungal flora in faeces. Clin Pharmacol Ther 10:675-680
39. Hofstra W, de Vries-Hospers HG, van der Waaij D (1979) Concentrations of nystatin in faeces after oral administration of various doses of nystatin. Infection 7:166-170
40. Hofstra W, de Vries-Hospers HG, van der Waaij D (1982) Concentrations of amphotericin B in faeces and blood of healthy volunteers after oral administration of various doses. Infection 10:233-277
41. Ramos B, Taylor N, Sarginson RE et al (2007) Enteral antimicrobials do not protect against acquisition and subsequent carriage of Staphylococcus aureus in a paediatric ICU using SDD. Epidemiol Infect [submitted for publication]
42. Walsh B, Salzmann M, Gaunt N et al (1985) Methicillin-resistant Staphylococcus aureus. Lancet II:219-220
43. Stoutenbeek CP, Miranda DR, van Saene HKF (1982) A new technique for infection prevention in the intensive care unit. Abstract, Proceedings of the 6th European Congress of Anaesthesiology. Anaesthesia: 56, abstract 98
44. van Saene JJM, Stoutenbeek CP, van Saene HKF (1992) Faecal endotoxin in human volunteers. Microb Ecol Health Dis 5:179-184
45. van Saene HKF, Stoutenbeek CP, Faber-Nijholt R et al (1992) Selective decontamination of the digestive tract contributes to the control of disseminated intra-vascular coagulation in severe liver impairment. J Pediatr Gastroenterol Nutr 4:436-442
46. van Saene JJM, Stoutenbeek CP, van Saene HKF et al (1996) Reduction of the intestinal endotoxin pool by three different SDD regimens in human volunteers. J Endotoxin Res 3:337-343

47. Greenfield S, Teres D, Bushnell LS et al (1973) Prevention of gram-negative bacillary pneumonia using aerosol polymyxin as prophylaxis. I. Effect on the colonization pattern of the upper respiratory tract of seriously ill patients. J Clin Invest 52:2935-2940
48. Klick JM, Du Moulin GC, Hedley-Whyte J et al (1975) Prevention of gram-negative bacillary pneumonia using polymyxin aerosol prophylaxis. II. Effect on the incidence of pneumonia in seriously ill patients. J Clin Invest 55:514-519
49. Feeley TW, Du Moulin GC, Hedley-Whyte J et al (1975) Aerosol polymyxin and pneumonia in seriously ill patients. N Engl J Med 293:471-475
50. Johanson WG (1989) Infection prevention by selective decontamination in intensive care. Intensive Care Med 15:417-419
51. Bodey GP (1981) Antibiotic prophylaxis in cancer patients: regimens of oral, nonabsorbable antibiotics for prevention of infection during induction of remission. Rev Infect Dis 3 [Suppl]:S259-S268
52. Jordan HV, De Paola PF (1974) Effect of a topically applied 3% vancomycin gel on Streptococcus mutans on different tooth surfaces. J Dent Res 53:115-120
53. Borthen L. Heimdahl A, Nord CE (1988) Effect of topical administration of vancomycin versus chlorhexidine on a-hemolytic streptococci in oral cavity. Oral Surg Oral Med Oral Pathol 66:304-309
54. de Vries-Hospers HG, van der Waaij D (1978) Amphotericin B concentrations in saliva after application of 2% amphotericin B in Orabase. Infection 6:3-15
55. Dever LL, Johanson WG (1993) An update on selective decontamination of the digestive tract. Curr Opin Infect Dis 6:744-750
56. Johanson WG, Seidenfeld JJ, de los Santos R et al (1988) Prevention of nosocomial pneumonia using topical and parenteral antimicrobial agents. Am Rev Respir Dis 137:265-272
57. Fine J, Frank H, Schweinburg F et al (1952) The bacterial factor in traumatic shock. Ann N Y Acad Sciences 55:429-445.
58. Ketchel SJ, Rodriguez V (1978) Acute infections in cancer patients. Semin Oncol 5:167-179
59. Rodriguez V, Whitecar JP, Bodey GP (1969) Therapy of infections with the combination of carbenicillin and gentamicin. Antimicrob Agents Chemother 9:386-390
60. Stoutenbeek CP (1989) The role of systemic antibiotic prophylaxis in infection prevention in intensive care by SDD. Infection 17:418-421
61. Alcock SR (1990) Short-term parenteral antibiotics used as a supplement to SDD regimens. Infection 13 [Suppl 1]:S14–S18
62. Kaiser AB (1986) Antimicrobial prophylaxis in surgery. N Engl J Med 315:1129-1138
63. Fox MA, Sarginson RE, Zandstra DF et al (2005) Comment on "Risk factors for late-onset ventilator-associated pneumonia in trauma patients receiving selective digestive decontamination" by Leone et al. Intensive Care Med 31:999
64. Stoutenbeek CP, van Saene HKF, Zandstra DF (1996) Prevention of multiple organ system failure by selective decontamination of the digestive tract in multiple trauma patients. In: Faist E, Baue AE, Schildberg FW (eds). The immune consequences of trauma, shock and sepsis-mechanisms and therapeutic approach. Lengerich: Pabst Science Publishers, pp 1055-1066
65. Krom RAF (1986) Liver transplantation at the Mayo clinic. Mayo Clin Proc 61:278-282
66. van der Waaij D, Sluiter HJ (1986) Luchtweginfecties bij patiënten in afdelingen voor intensieve behandeling; pathogenese en preventie. Ned Tijdschr Geneeskd 130:854-858
67. van Saene HKF, Stoutenbeek CP (1986) Luchtweginfecties bij patiënten in afdelingen voor intensieve behandeling; pathogenese en preventie. Ned Tijdschr Geneeskd 130:1291
68. van der Waaij D (1987) Selective decontamination of the digestive tract in surgical intensive care units. Intensive Care World 4:44-47
69. Miranda DR, Langrehr D (1988) The control of Gram-negative bacterial infection in the ICU. (Recent advances in critical care medicine, no 3) Churchill Livingstone, Edinburgh, pp 135-157
70. Hermans WF. Onder professoren (1975) Tweede druk Amsterdam De Bezige Bij ISBN 90 234 6036 7

71. Abele-Horn M, Dauber A, Bauernfeind A et al (1997) Decrease in nosocomial pneumonia in ventilated patients by selective oropharyngeal decontamination (SOD). Intensive Care Med 23:187-195
72. Aerdts SJ, van Dalen R, Clasener HA et al (1991) Antibiotic prophylaxis of respiratory tract infection in mechanically ventilated patients. A prospective, blinded, randomized trial of the effect of a novel regimen. Chest 100:783-791
73. Arnow PM, Carandang GC, Zabner R et al (1996) Randomized controlled trial of selective bowel decontamination for prevention of infections following liver transplantation. Clin Infect Dis 22:997-1003
74. Barret JP, Jeschke MG, Herndon DN (2001) Selective decontamination of the digestive tract in severely burned pediatric patients. Burns 27:439-445
75. Bergmans DC, Bonten MJ, Gaillard CA et al (2001) Prevention of ventilator-associated pneumonia by oral decontamination: a prospective, randomized, double-blind, placebo-controlled study. Am J Respir Crit Care Med 164:382-388
76. Bion JF, Badger I, Crosby HA et al (1994) Selective decontamination of the digestive tract reduces gram-negative pulmonary colonization but not systemic endotoxemia in patients undergoing elective liver transplantation. Crit Care Med 22:40-49
77. Blair P, Rowlands BJ, Lowry K et al (1991) Selective decontamination of the digestive tract: a stratified, randomized, prospective study in a mixed intensive care unit. Surgery 110:303-309
78. Boland JP, Sadler DL, Stewart W et al (1991) Reduction of nosocomial respiratory infections in multiple trauma patients requiring mechanical ventilation by selective parenteral and enteral antisepsis regimen (SPEAR) in the intensive care. Seventeenth international congress of chemotherapy Berlin, 1991, abstract 0465
79. Bouter H, Schippers EF, Luelmo SA et al (2002) No effect of preoperative selective gut decontamination on endotoxemia and cytokine activation during cardiopulmonary bypass: a randomized, placebo-controlled study. Crit Care Med 30:38-43
80. Brun-Buisson C, Legrand P, Rauss A et al (1989) Intestinal decontamination for control of nosocomial multi-resistant gram-negative bacilli. Ann Intern Med 110:873-881
81. de la Cal MA, Cerda E, Garcia-Hierro P et al (2005) Survival benefit in critically ill burned patients receiving selective decontamination of the digestive tract: a randomized, placebo controlled, double blind trial. Ann Surg 241:424-430
82. Camus C, Bellissant E, Sebille V et al (2005) Prevention of acquired infections in intubated patients with the combination of two decontamination regimens. Crit Care Med 33:307-314
83. Cerra FB, Maddaus MA, Dunn DL et al (1992) Selective gut decontamination reduces nosocomial infections and length of stay but not mortality or organ failure in surgical intensive care unit patients. Arch Surg 127:163-169
84. Cockerill FR, III, Muller SR, Anhalt JP et al (1992) Prevention of infection in critically ill patients by selective decontamination of the digestive tract. Ann Intern Med 117:545-553
85. Ferrer M, Torres A, Gonzalez J et al (1994) Utility of selective digestive decontamination in mechanically ventilated patients. Ann Intern Med 120:389-395
86. Finch RG, Tomlinson P, Holliday M et al (1991) Selective decontamination of the digestive tract (SDD) in the prevention of secondary sepsis in a medical/surgical intensive care unit. Seventeenth International Congress of Chemotherapy, Berlin, 1991, abstract 0471
87. Flaherty J, Nathan C, Kabins SA et al (1990) Pilot trial of selective decontamination for prevention of bacterial infection in an intensive care unit. J Infect Dis 162:1393-1397
88. Gastinne H, Wolff M, Delatour F et al (1992) A controlled trial in intensive care units of selective decontamination of the digestive tract with non-absorbable antibiotics. N Engl J Med 326:594-599
89. Gaussorgues P, Salord F, Sirodot M et al (1991) Efficacité de la décontamination digestive sur la survenue des bactériémies nosocomiales chez les patients sous ventilation méchanique et recevant des betamimétiques. Réanimation Soins Intensifs Médecin d'Urgence 7:169-174
90. Georges B, Mazerolles M, Decun J-F, Rouge P et al (1994) Décontamination digestive sélective résultats d'une étude chez polytraumatisés. Réanimation Urgence 3:621-627

91. Gosney M, Martin MV, Wright AE (2006) The role of selective decontamination of the digestive tract in acute stroke. Age Aging 35:42-47
92. Hammond JM, Potgieter PD, Saunders GL et al (1992) Double-blind study of selective decontamination of the digestive tract in intensive care. Lancet 340:5-9
93. Hellinger WC, Yao JD, Alvarez S et al (2002) A randomized, prospective, double-blinded evaluation of selective bowel decontamination in liver transplantation. Transplantation 73:1904-1909
94. Jacobs S, Foweraker JE, Roberts SE (1992) Effectiveness of selective decontamination of the digestive tract (SDD) in an ICU with a policy encouraging a low gastric pH. Clin Intensive Care 3:52-58
95. de Jonge E, Schultz MJ, Spanjaard L et al (2003) Effects of selective decontamination of digestive tract on mortality and acquisition of resistant bacteria in intensive care: a randomised controlled trial. Lancet 362:1011-1016
96. Kerver AJH, Rommes JH, Mevissen-Verhage EAE et al (1988) Prevention of colonization and infection in critically ill patients: a prospective randomized study. Crit Care Med 16:1087-1093
97. Korinek AM, Laisne MJ, Nicolas MH et al (1993) Selective decontamination of the digestive tract in neurosurgical intensive care unit patients: a double-blind, randomized, placebo-controlled study. Crit Care Med 21:1466-1473
98. Krueger WA, Lenhart FP, Neeser G et al (2002) Influence of combined intravenous and topical antibiotic prophylaxis on the incidence of infections, organ dysfunctions, and mortality in critically ill surgical patients: A prospective, stratified, randomized, double-blind, placebo-controlled clinical trial. Am J Respir Crit Care Med 166:1029-1037
99. Laggner AN, Tryba M, Georgopoulos A et al (1994) Oropharyngeal decontamination with gentamicin for long-term ventilated patients on stress ulcer prophylaxis with sucralfate? Wien Klin Wochenschr 106:15-19
100. Lingnau W, Berger J, Javorsky F et al (1997) Selective intestinal decontamination in multiple trauma patients: prospective, controlled trial. J Trauma 42:687-694
101. Luiten EJT, Hop WCJ, Lange JF et al (1995) Controlled clinical trial of selective decontamination for the treatment of severe acute pancreatitis. Ann Surg 222:57-65
102. Martinez-Pellus AE, Merino P, Bru M et al (1993) Can selective digestive decontamination avoid the endotoxemia and cytokine activation promoted by cardiopulmonary bypass? Crit Care Med 21:1684-1691
103. Martinez-Pellus AE, Merino P, Bru M et al (1997) Endogenous endotoxemia of intestinal origin during cardiopulmonary bypass. Role of type of flow and protective effect of selective digestive decontamination. Intensive Care Med 23:1251-1257
104. Palomar M, Alvarez-Lerma F, Jorda R et al for the Catalan study group of nosocomial pneumonia prevention (1997) Prevention of nosocomial pneumonia in mechanically ventilated patients: selective decontamination versus sucralfate. Clin Intensive Care 8:228-235
105. Pneumatikos I, Koulouras V, Nathanail C et al (2002) Selective decontamination of subglottic area in mechanically ventilated patients with multiple trauma. Intensive Care Med 28:432-437
106. Pugin J, Auckenthaler R, Lew DP et al (1991) Oropharyngeal decontamination decreases incidence of ventilator- associated pneumonia. A randomized, placebo-controlled, double-blind clinical trial. JAMA 265:2704-2710
107. Quinio B, Albanese J, Bues-Charbit M et al (1996) Selective decontamination of the digestive tract in multiple trauma patients. A prospective, double-blind, randomized, placebo-controlled study. Chest 109:765-772
108. Rayes N, Seehofer D, Hansen S et al (2002) Early enteral supply of Lactobacillus and fibre versus selective bowel decontamination: A controlled trial in liver transplant recipients. Transplantation 74:123-128
109. Rocha LA, Martin MJ, Pita S et al (1992) Prevention of nosocomial infections in critically ill patients by selective decontamination of the digestive tract. A randomised, double blind, placebo controlled study. Intensive Care Med 18:398-404

110. Rodriguez-Roldan JM, Altuna-Cuesta A, Lopez A et al (1990) Prevention of nosocomial lung infection in ventilated patients: use of an antimicrobial pharyngeal nonabsorbable paste. Crit Care Med 18:1239-1242
111. Rolando N, Gimson A, Wade J et al (1993) Prospective controlled trial of selective parenteral and enteral antimicrobial regimen in fulminant liver failure. Hepatology 17:196-201
112. Rolando N, Wade JJ, Stangou A, Gimson AE et al (1996) Prospective study comparing the efficacy of prophylactic parenteral antimicrobials, with or without enteral decontamination, in patients with acute liver failure. Liver Transpl Surg 2:8-13
113. Ruza F, Alvarado F, Herruzo R et al (1998) Prevention of nosocomial infection in a pediatric intensive care unit (PICU) through the use of selective digestive decontamination. Eur J Epidemiol 14:719-727
114. Sanchez GM, Cambronero Galache JA et al (1998) Effectiveness and cost of selective decontamination of the digestive tract in critically ill intubated patients. A randomized, double-blind, placebo-controlled, multicenter trial. Am J Respir Crit Care Med 158:908-916
115. Schardey HM, Joosten U, Finke U et al (1997) The prevention of anastomotic leakage after total gastrectomy with local decontamination. A prospective, randomized, double-blind, placebo- controlled multicenter trial. Ann Surg 225:172-180
116. Smith SD, Jackson RJ, Hannakan CJ et al (1993) Selective decontamination in pediatric liver transplants. A randomized prospective study. Transplantation 55:1306-1309
117. Stoutenbeek CP, van Saene HKF, Zandstra DF (1996) Prevention of multiple organ system failure by selective decontamination of the digestive tract in multiple trauma patients. In: Faist EBAE, Schildberg FW (eds) Immune consequences of trauma, shock and sepsis. Lengerich: Pabst Science Publishers, pp 1055-1066.
118. Stoutenbeek CP, van Saene HKF, Little RA et al (2007) The effect of selective decontamination of the digestive tract on mortality in multiple trauma patients. Intensive Care Med 33:261-270
119. Tetteroo GW, Wagenvoort JH, Castelein A et al (1990) Selective decontamination to reduce gram-negative colonization and infections after oesophageal resection. Lancet 335:704-707
120. Ulrich C, Harinck-de Weerd JE, Bakker NC et al (1989) Selective decontamination of the digestive tract with norfloxacin in the prevention of ICU-acquired infections: a prospective, randomized study. Intensive Care Med 15:424-431
121. Unertl K, Ruckdeschel G, Selbmann HK et al (1987) Prevention of colonization and respiratory infections in long-term ventilated patients by local antimicrobial prophylaxis. Intensive Care Med 13:106-113
122. Verwaest C, Verhaegen J, Ferdinande P et al (1997) Randomized controlled trial of selective digestive decontamination in 600 mechanically ventilated patients in a multi-disciplinary intensive care unit. Crit Care Med 25:63-71
123. Wiener J, Itokazu G, Nathan C et al (1995) A randomized, double-blind, placebo controlled trial of selective digestive decontamination in a medical, surgical intensive care unit. Clin Infect Dis 20:861-867
124. Winter R, Humphreys H, Pick A et al (1992) A controlled trial of selective decontamination of the digestive tract in intensive care and its effect on nosocomial infection. J Antimicrob Chemother 30:73-87
125. Zobel G, Kuttnig M, Grubbauer HM et al (1991) Reduction of colonization and infection rate during pediatric intensive care by selective decontamination of the digestive tract. Crit Care Med 19:1242-1246
126. Zwaveling JH, Maring JK, Klompmaker IJ et al (2002) Selective decontamination of the digestive tract to prevent postoperative infection: a randomized placebo-controlled trial in liver transplant patients. Crit Care Med 30:1204-1209
127. McA Ledingham I, Alcock SR, Eastaway AT et al (1988) Triple regimen of selective decontamination of the digestive tract, systemic cefotaxime, and microbiological surveillance for prevention of acquired infection in intensive care. Lancet I:785-790
128. Hünefeld G (1989) Selective digestive decolonization in long-term ventilated surgical patients. Anesthesiol Reanim 14:131-153

129. Konrad F, Schwalbe B, Heeg K et al (1989) Frequency of bacterial colonization and respiratory tract infections and resistance behaviour in patients subjected to long-term ventilated patients with selective decontamination of the digestive tract. Anaesthesist 38:99-109
130. Nardi G, Valentinis U, Bartaletti R et al (1990) Effectiveness of topic selective digestive decontamination, without any systemic antibiotic prophylaxis, in the prevention of pulmonary infections in ICU patients. Minerva Anestesiol 56:19-26
131. Sydow M, Burchardi H, Crozier TA et al (1990) Influence of selective decontamination on nosocomial infections, their causative agents and resistance to antibiotics in long-term intubated intensive care patients. Anaesth Intensivther Notfallmed 25:416-423
132. Godard J, Guillaume C, Reverdy ME et al (1990) Intestinal decontamination in a polyvalent ICU. Intensive Care Med 16:307-311
133. Hartenauer U, Thulig B, Diemer W et al (1991) Effect of selective flora suppression on colonization, infection, and mortality in critically ill patients: A one-year prospective consecutive study. Crit Care Med 19:463-473
134. Fox MA, Peterson S, Fabri BM et al (1991) Selective decontamination of the digestive tract in cardiac surgical patients. Crit Care Med 19:1486-1490
135. McClelland P, Murray AE, Williams PS et al (1990) Reducing sepsis in severe combined acute renal and respiratory failure by selective decontamination of the digestive tract. Crit Care Med 18:935-939
136. McClelland P, Murray A, Yagoob M et al (1992) Prevention of bacterial infection and sepsis in acute severe pancreatitis. Ann R Coll Surg Engl 74:329-334
137. Mackie DP, van Hertum WAJ, Schumburg T et al (1992) Prevention of infection in burns: preliminary experience with selective decontamination of the digestive tract in patients with extensive injuries. J Trauma 32:570-575
138. Lipman J, Klugman K and The Baragwanath SDD Study Group (1994) A modified form of selective decontamination of the digestive tract (m SDD) in a multi-disciplinary adult and paediatric intensive care unit. Clin Intensive Care 5: Suppl 70
139. Riedl SE, Peter B, Geiss HK et al (2001) Microbiological and clinical effect of selective bowel decontamination trans thoracic resections of the carcinoma of the oesophagus and cardia. Chirurg 72:1160-1170
140. Aitchison JM, van den Ende J, van Rensburg HCG et al (1991) Prospective study of the selective parenteral and enteral antibiotic regimen (SPEAR) in critically ill surgical patients. Seventeenth International Congress of Chemotherapy, abstract 0460
141. Dobb GJ, Boyle SM (1999) The effect of selective decontamination of the digestive tract (SDD) on nosocomial pneumonia and mortality in an Australian intensive care unit. Clinical intensive care poster abstract 1, 12th International Symposium on Intensive Care and Emergency Medicine
142. Parra ML, Arias S, de la Cal MA et al (2002) Effect of selective digestive decontamination on the nosocomial infection and multi-resistant micro-organisms incidence in critically ill patients. Med Clin (Barc) 118:361-364
143. Meynaar IA, van den Elzakker E, Visser C et al (2005) Cefazolin as parenteral component of selective digestive decontamination. European Congress of Intensive Care Medicine, Amsterdam. Intensive Care Med 31:S28
144. Selective Decontamination of the Digestive Tract Trialists' Collaborative Group (1993) Meta-analysis of randomised controlled trials of selective decontamination of the digestive tract. BMJ 307:525-532
145. Heyland DK, Cook DJ, Jaeschke R et al (1994) Selective decontamination of the digestive tract: an overview. Chest 105:1221-1229
146. Kollef M (1994) The role of selective digestive tract decontamination on mortality and respiratory tract infections. A meta-analysis. Chest 105:1101-1108
147. D'Amico R, Pifferi S, Leonetti C et al (1998) Effectiveness of antibiotic prophylaxis in critically ill adult patients: systematic review of randomised controlled trials. BMJ 316:1275-1285
148. Nathens AB, Marshall JC (1999) Selective decontamination of the digestive tract in surgical patients. A systematic review of the evidence. Arch Surg 134:170-176

149. Redman R, Ludington E, Crocker M et al and the VAP Advisory Group (2001) Analysis of respiratory and non-respiratory infections in published trials of selective digestive decontamination. Intensive Care Med 27 [Suppl 1]: S285
150. Liberati A, D'Amico R, Pifferi S et al (2004) Antibiotic prophylaxis to reduce respiratory tract infections and mortality in adults receiving intensive care. (Cochrane review; The Cochrane Library, Issue 1) Chichester, UK: Wiley
151. Safdar N, Said A, Lucey MR (2004) The role of selective decontamination for reducing infection in patients undergoing liver transplant: a systematic review and meta-analysis. Liver Transpl 10:817-827
152. Silvestri L, van Saene HKF, Milanese M et al (2005) Impact of selective decontamination of the digestive tract on fungal carriage and infection : systematic review of randomised controlled trials. Intensive Care Med 31:898-910
153. Silvestri L, van Saene HKF, Milanese M et al (2007) Selective decontamination of the digestive tract reduces bacterial bloodstream infection and mortality: systematic review of randomised, controlled trials. J Hosp Infect 65:187-203
154. Vandenbroucke-Grauls CMJE, Vandenbroucke JP (1991) Effect of selective decontamination of the digestive tract on respiratory tract infections and mortality in the intensive care unit. Lancet 338:859-863
155. Hurley JC (1995) Prophylaxis with enteral antibiotics in ventilated patients: selective decontamination or selective cross-infection? Antimicrob Agents Chemother 39:941-947
156. van Nieuwenhoven CA, Buskens E, van Thiel EA et al (2001) Relationship between methodological trial quality and the effects of selective digestive decontamination on pneumonia and mortality in critically ill patients. JAMA 286:335-340
157. Ebner W, Kropec-Hübner A, Daschner FD (2000) Bacterial resistance and overgrowth due to selective decontamination of the digestive tract. Eur J Clin Microbiol Infect Dis 19:243-247
158. Rommes JH, Zandstra DF, van Saene HKF (1999) Selective decontamination of the digestive tract reduces mortality in intensive care patients. Ned Tijdschr Geneeskd 143:602-606
159. Kerver AJH, Rommes JH, Mevissen-Verhage EAE et al (1987) Colonisation and infection in surgical intensive care patients–a prospective year. Intensive Care Med 13:347-351
160. van Furth R (1995) Infektieziekten–verleden en heden. In: van Es JC, Kleeman JN, de Leeuw PW et al (eds) Medisch Jaar 1995. Bohn, Houten Hst 15; pp 226-245
161. Verhoef J, Verhaege EAE, Visser MR (1993) A decade of experience with selective decontamination of the digestive tract as prophylaxis for infections in patients in the intensive care unit: what have we learned? Clin Infect Dis 17:1047-1054
162. Bonten MJM (2003) Prevention of hospital-acquired pneumonia: European perspective. Infect Dis Clin N Am 17:773-784
163. de la Cal MA, Cerda E, Garcia-Hierro P et al (2001) Pneumonia in patients with severe burns. A classification according to the concept of the carrier state. Chest 119:1160-1165
164. de la Cal MA, Cerda E, van Saene HKF et al (2004) Effectiveness and safety of enteral vancomycin to control endemicity of methicillin-resistant Staphylococcus aureus in a medical/surgical intensive care. J Hosp Infect 56:175-183
165. Cerdá E, Abella A, de la Cal MA et al (2007) Enteral vancomycin controls methicillin-resistant Staphylococcus aureus endemicity in an intensive care burn unit: a 9-year prospective study. Ann Surg 245:397-407
166. Gilston A (1991) Down with dogma. Intensive Crit Care Dig 10:36
167. Atkinson SW, Bihari DJ (1993) Selective decontamination of the gut. Does not affect survival in intensive care units. BMJ 306:286-287
168. Sanderson PJ (1989) Selective decontamination of the digestive tract. Value in intensive care units not proved. BMJ 299:1413-1414
169. Webb CH (2000) Selective decontamination of the digestive tract, SDD: a commentary. J Hosp Infect 46:106-109
170. Conscience G, Misset B, Carlet J (1991) SDD in intensive care units: review of trials and future prospects. La letter de l'infectiologue 6:635-639

171. Brun-Buisson C (1993) Risk factors for nosocomial pneumonia. In: Vincent JL (ed) Yearbook of intensive care and emergency medicine 1993. Springer, Berlin; pp 273-280
172. Leone M, Albanese J, Antonini F et al (2003) Long-term (6-year) effect of selective digestive decontamination on antimicrobial resistance in intensive care, multiple-trauma patients. Crit Care Med 31:2090-2095
173. Hamer DH, Barza M (1993) Prevention of hospital-acquired pneumonia in critically ill patients. Antimicrob Agents Chemother 37:931-938
174. Bigatello LM, Zapol WM (1996) New approaches to acute lung injury. Br J Anaesth 77:99-109
175. Mayhall CG (1997) Nosocomial pneumonia. Diagnosis and prevention. Infect Dis Clin North Am 11:427-457.
176. Kollef MH (1999) The prevention of ventilator-associated pneumonia. N Engl J Med 340:627-634
177. Sadfar N, Maki DG (2002) The commonality of risk factors for nosocomial colonisation and infection with antimicrobial-resistant Staphylococcus aureus, Enterococcus, Gram-negative bacilli, Clostridium difficile and Candida. Ann Intern Med 136:834-844
178. Silvestri L, van Saene HKF, Milanese M et al (2004) Prevention of MRSA pneumonia by oral vancomycin decontamination: a randomised trial. Eur Respir J 23:921-926
179. Baltussen A, Kindler CH (2004) Citation classics in critical care medicine. Intensive Care Med 30:902-910
180. Liberati A, D'Amico R, Brazzi L et al (2001) Influence of methodological quality on study conclusions. JAMA 286:2544-2547
181. Bonten MJM (2003) Prevention of hospital-acquired pneumonia: European perspective. Infect Dis Clin North Am 17:773-784
182. Bonten MJM (2002) Strategies for prevention of hospital-acquired pneumonia: oral and selective decontamination of the gastro-intestinal tract. Semin Respir Crit Care Med 23:481-488
183. van Saene HKF, Stoutenbeek CP, Lawin P, McA Ledingham I (eds) (1989) Infection control by selective decontamination. (Update in intensive care and emergency medicine, no 7) Springer, Berlin
184. Carlet J, Artigas A, Bihari D et al (1992) Consensus Conference Report. The first European Consensus Conference in Intensive Care Medicine. Intensive Care Med 18:180-188
185. van Saene HKF, Silvestri L, de la Cal MA (eds). (1998) Infection control in the intensive care unit, 1st edn. (Topics in anaesthesia and critical care) Springer-Verlag Italia, Milan
186. van Saene HKF, Silvestri L, de la Cal MA (eds) (2005) Infection control in the intensive care unit, 2nd edn. (Topics in anaesthesia and critical care) Springer-Verlag Italia, Milan
187. Sacket DL (2000) The sins of expertness and a proposal for redemption. BMJ 320:1283
188. Unertl K (1986) Nosocomiale bakterielle Infektionen der Respirationstraktes bei beatmeten Patienten. PhD thesis, Ludwig Maximilian University, Munich
189. Stoutenbeek CP (1987) Infection prevention in intensive care. Infection prevention in multiple trauma patients by selective decontamination of the digestive tract (SDD). PhD thesis, Groningen
190. Kerver AJH (1988) Nosocomial infections and infection prevention in surgical intensive care patients. Thesis, Faculty of Medicine, University of Utrecht
191. Aerdts SJA (1989) Prevention of lower respiratory infection in mechanically ventilated patients. PhD thesis, Faculty of Medicine, University of Maastricht
192. van Nieuwenhoven CA (2007) Prevention of ventilator-associated pneumonia: making a difference? PhD Thesis, Faculty of Medicine, University of Maastricht, The Netherlands
193. Grundling M (1992) Pneumonieprophylaxe bei langzeitbeatmeten Intensivtherapiepatienten durch selektive Darmdekontamination. PhD Thesis, Faculty of Medicine, University of Greifswald, Germany
194. Spijkervet FKL (1989) Irradiation mucositis and oral flora. Reduction of mucositis by selective elimination of oral flora. PhD thesis, Faculty of Medicine, University of Groningen
195. van Saene JJM (1990) Colonic delivery of polymyxin E and four quinolones for flora suppression. Thesis, Faculty of Sciences, University of Groningen

196. Vollaard EJ (1991) The concept of colonization resistance. A study of the influence of antimicrobial agents on the aerobic flora of the bowel. PhD thesis, Faculty of Medicine & Dentistry, University of Nijmegen
197. Verhaegen J (1992) Randomized study of selective digestive decontamination on colonization and prevention of infections in mechanically ventilated patients in the ICU. PhD thesis, Faculty of Medicine, University of Leuven
198. Manson WL (1992) Microbiological studies in burns. PhD thesis, Faculty of Medicine, Rijksuniversiteit Groningen
199. van Bebber IPT (1992) An experimental model of the adult respiratory distress syndrome and multiple organ failure: zymosan induced generalized inflammation. Thesis, Faculty of Medicine, University of Nijmegen
200. Ameen ASM (1993) Microbiological studies in mice of intestinal decontamination regimens. PhD Thesis, Faculty of Medicine, University of Glasgow
201. Tetteroo GWM (1993) Infection prevention in the surgical intensive care unit using selective decontamination. Thesis, Faculty of Medicine, University of Rotterdam
202. Bonten MJM (1994) The role of colonization of the upper intestinal tract in the pathogenesis of ventilator-associated pneumonia. Thesis, Rijksuniversiteit Maastricht
203. Hammond JMJ (1993) Nosocomial infection in intensive care. PhD thesis, Faculty of Medicine, University of Cape Town, South Africa
204. Blair PHB (1994) The clinical and microbiological effects of selective decontamination of the digestive tract in a mixed intensive care unit. MD thesis, Faculty of Medicine, The Queen's University of Belfast
205. Luiten EJT (1998) Severe acute pancreatitis and selective decontamination. PhD thesis, Erasmus University Rotterdam
206. Bergmans DCJJ (1999) Ventilator-associated pneumonia; studies on pathogenesis, diagnosis and prevention. PhD thesis, Faculty of Medicine, University of Maastricht
207. van der Voort PHJ (1999) Helicobacter pylori in the critically ill. Thesis, Faculty of Medicine, University of Amsterdam
208. Conraads VM (2002) Inflammation and chronic heart failure determinants and modulation. PhD thesis, Faculty of Medicine, University of Antwerp
209. Morar P (2003) Lower airway infections in tracheotomised children: magnitude and control of the exogenous infection. MD thesis, Faculty of Medicine, University of Liverpool
210. Fagon JY, Chastre J, Wolff M et al (2000) Invasive and non-invasive strategies for management of suspected ventilator-associated pneumonia: a randomised trial. Ann Intern Med 132:621-630
211. Gastinne H, Wolff M, Lachatre G et al (1992) Antibiotic levels in bronchial tree and in serum during selective digestive decontamination. Intensive Care Med 17:215-218
212. Bonten MJM, Kullberg BJ, Filius PMG (2001) Optimizing antibiotics policy in the Netherlands. VI SWAB advice: no selective decontamination of IC patients on mechanical ventilation. Ned Tijdschr Geneeskd 145:353-357
213. Koeman M, van der Ven AJAM, Hak E et al (2006) Oral decontamination with chlorhexidine reduces the incidence of ventilator-associated pneumonia. Am J Respir Crit Care Med 173:1348-1355
214. Bonten JMJ, van Tiel FH, van der Geest S et al (1993) Enterococcus faecalis pneumonia complicating topical antimicrobial prophylaxis. N Engl J Med 328:209-210
215. Nixon JR, Nielsen MS (2000) Selective decontamination of the digestive tract–current national practice. Br J Anaesth 84:682P-683P
216. Bogaards MJ (2001) An inventarisation of the products. Selective digestive decontamination in the Netherlands. Pharm Weekdl 136:706-712
217. Vincent JL (1999) Prevention of nosocomial bacterial pneumonia. Thorax 54:544-549
218. Aarts MA, Marshall JC (2002) In defense of evidence. Am J Respir Crit Care Med 166:1014-1015
219. Farr BM (2000) Reasons for non-compliance with infection control guidelines. Infect Control Hosp Epidemiol 21:411-416

220. Antman EM, Lau J, Kupeluick B et al (1992) A comparison of results on meta-analyses of randomized controlled trials and recommendations of clinical experts. JAMA 268:240-248
221. Kollef MH (1996) Long-term effects of selective decontamination on antimicrobial resistance. Crit Care Med 24:177-178
222. Wazana A (2000) Physicians and the pharmaceutical industry. Is a gift ever just a gift? JAMA 285:373-386
223. Garattini S, Liberati A (2000) The risk of bias from omitted research. Evidence must be independently sought and free of economic interests. BMJ 321:845-846
224. van Saene HKF, Silvestri L, de la Cal MA et al (2006) Selective decontamination of the digestive tract reduces lower airway and bloodstream infection and mortality and prevents emergence of antimicrobial resistance. Microbes Infect 8:953-954
225. Silvestri L, van Saene HKF (2006) Selective decontamination of the digestive tract does not increase resistance in critically ill patients: evidence from randomized controlled trials. Crit Care Med 34:2027-2029
226. Damjanovic V, van Saene HKF (2005) Microbial mutation as a source of polyclonality in the gut of the critically ill. J Hosp Infect 59:374-375
227. Torres A, Carlet J (2001) European task force on ventilator-associated pneumonia. Ventilator-associated pneumonia. Eur Respir J 17:1034-1045
228. NVIC guidelines for the prevention of pneumonia during mechanical ventilation. Richtlijn. Het voorkomen van bacteriele longontstreking en stenfte tijdens beademing. (2006) Neth J Crit Care 10:38-52
229. British Society of Antimicrobial Chemotherapy [BSAC]. Hospital acquired pneumonia [HAP]: Considered judgement. Consultation Document, 2005
230. University of California at San Francisco, Stanford University Evidence-based Practice Center (2001) Making healthcare safer: a critical analysis of patient safety practice. www.ahrg.gov/clinic/ptsafety

Chapter 2
The Concept of SDD

Hans J. Rommes

Introduction

Selective decontamination of the digestive tract (SDD) is a prophylactic strategy designed to minimise the infection-related morbidity and mortality in patients admitted to the intensive care unit (ICU) [1, 2]. Effective and safe use of the SDD method of infection prevention requires a full understanding of this strategy and of its aims and limitations. The concept of SDD is based on three pillars: (1) 14 (15 if MRSA is included) microorganisms are responsible for over 95% of infections in ICU patients; (2) infections in ICU patients are classified into primary endogenous, secondary endogenous and exogenous infections; and (3) effective and safe infection control of the three types of infection requires the full four-component SDD protocol. This chapter describes the principles behind the SDD concept, the four components of the SDD strategy, and the main differences between traditional and SDD microbiology.

The Fourteen Bacteria

Traditionally, microorganisms are classified according to their biochemical properties, such as whether they are gram-positive or gram-negative, and their morphological properties, i.e. whether they are rods or cocci. Unfortunately, there is no relation between their morphological and biochemical properties and their pathogenicity. For instance, the mortality of septicaemia caused by community-acquired gram-positive or gram-negative microorganisms is similar, at 29.2% and 26.8%, respectively [3]. Alternatively, mortality rates are quite different amongst patients with respiratory tract infections attributable to *H. influenzae* and *Pseudomonas aeruginosa*, although both are aerobic gram-negative bacilli (AGNB) [4]. Microorganisms differ in their pathogenicity. The clinical impact of this variance in virulence is illustrated by the observation

P.H.J. van der Voort, H.K.F. van Saene (eds.) *Selective Digestive Tract Decontamination in Intensive Care Medicine.*

that although 99% of ICU patients are carriers of enterococci in high concentrations in the gut, infection seldom occurs as a result of this microorganism. Conversely, 30–40 % of ICU patients who carry AGNB such as *Pseudomonas aeruginosa* or *Klebsiella spp.* in the oropharynx or gut develop an infection caused by these microorganisms [5]. Intensivists are interested in the clinical relevance of the presence of a microorganism in a diagnostic sample. Does isolation of enterococci in the secretions of the lower airways have the same clinical importance as isolation of *Ps. aeruginosa* from the same site? Should a patient with clinical signs of an infection and coagulase-negative staphylococci in the tracheal aspirate be treated with vancomycin? From a clinical point of view, a classification based on the pathogenicity of microorganisms is more appropriate than the traditional classification based on the Gram stain. Leonard et al. introduced a formula, the Intrinsic Pathogenicity Index (IPI), to indicate the capacity of a microorganism to cause infection [6]. For a microorganism, species x, causing infection in ICU patients, the IPI is the ratio between the number of patients infected by x and the number of patients carrying species x in the throat/gut.

$$\text{IPI} = \frac{\text{Number of patients infected by species } x}{\text{Number of patients carrying species } x \text{ in throat/gut}}$$

The range of the IPI is 0–1. Carriage of a microorganism with an IPI close to 0 will seldom be followed by an infection. Examples of these low-virulence microorganisms are anaerobes, coagulase-negative staphylococci and enterococci (Table 2.1). Infections with low-level pathogens occur only in special circumstances, such as hypoxia in necrotic tissue and disruption of the integrity of the skin in the case of a central venous or arterial line. Generally, these infections are easy to treat by drainage or removal of the plastic catheter. An IPI approaching 1 denotes a highly virulent microorganism such as *N. meningitidis* or *S. pyogenes*. Carriage or colonisation by such a high pathogenic microorganism nearly always leads to infection. Infections caused by high-level pathogens are characterised by a fulminant course and are generally easily recognised by an experienced intensivist. These important infections, which cause serious morbidity and mortality, are typically community acquired.

The ICU infection problem is related to potentially pathogenic microoorganisms (PPMs) with an IPI ranging from 0.3 to 0.4. There are 14 (15 including MRSA) PPMs, 6 'community' PPMs and 8 'hospital' PPMs. Healthy people carry only the normal 'community' PPMs besides their indigenous flora, while chronic underlying disease is associated with abnormal carriage of 'hospital' PPM [7, 8].

Table 2.1 Pathogenicity of microorganisms (MRSA, methicillin-resistant *Staphylococcus aureus;* IPI, Intrinsic Pathogenicity Index)

Intrinsic pathogenicity		Site of carriage	Microorganism	Flora
Low pathogenic microorganisms IPI = 0.01	Indigenous flora	Throat	*Peptostreptococci*, *Veillonella* spp., *Streptococcus viridans*	Normal
		Gut	*Bacteroides* spp., *Clostridium* spp., *enterococci*, *E. coli*	
		Vagina	*Peptostreptococci*, *Bacteroides* spp., *lactobacilli*, *Propionibacterium acnes*	
		Skin	Coagulase-negative staphylococci	
Potentially pathogenic microorganisms (PPMs) IPI = 0.3–0.6	'Community' PPM	Throat	*S. pneumoniae*, *H. influenzae*, *M. catarrhalis*, *S. aureus*, *Candida* spp.	Normal
		Gut	*E. coli*, *S. aureus*, *Candida* spp.	
	'Hospital' PPM	Throat and gut	*Klebsiella*, *Proteus*, *Morganella*, *Enterobacter*, *Citrobacter*, *Serratia*, *Pseudomonas*, *Acinetobacter* spp., MRSA	Abnormal
Highly pathogenic microorganisms IPI = 0.9–1.0	'Epidemic' microorganisms	Throat	*Neisseria meningitidis*	Abnormal
		Gut	*Salmonella* spp	

The Three Types of Infection

Three types of infection occur in the ICU: exogenous infections, primary endogenous infections and secondary endogenous infections (Table 2.2) [9].

Exogenous infections are caused by PPMs that are not carried by the patient in the throat and/or gut, but are suddenly isolated from diagnostic samples, e.g. lower airway secretions, urine, wound fluid or blood (Fig. 2.1). Exogenous infections are typically caused by 'hospital' PPM and can occur at any time throughout the treatment in the ICU. *Acinetobacter* spp. and *Pseudomonas* spp. such as

Table 2.2 Classification of ICU infections

Classification based on carrier status	Definition	Microorganisms	Onset
Exogenous infection	The causative PPM is introduced directly into the sterile internal organ without previous carriage	'Hospital' PPM	Any time during ICU treatment
Primary endogenous infection	Caused by PPM carried in throat and/or gut on admission	'Community' and 'hospital' PPM	Generally within 1 week of admission
Secondary endogenous infection	Caused by PPM not carried in throat and/or gut on admission. The PPM is acquired during ICU stay, causing carriage, colonisation and infection	'Hospital' PPM	Generally after 1 week in the ICU

Stenotrophomonas maltophilia are well recognised PPMs causing exogenous infections. These PPMs are transmitted via the hands of carers from one patient-carrier directly into the lower airways, bladder or wound of another patient, or are blown into the airways via contaminated ventilators, temperature probes in the ventilator circuit and heat and moisture exchangers. Numerous sources of exogenous infections are described. Despite infection control measures the incidence of exogenous infections is substantial. Recent cohort studies showed that in 15–20% of the infections in ICU patients the pathogenesis is exogenous [10, 11].

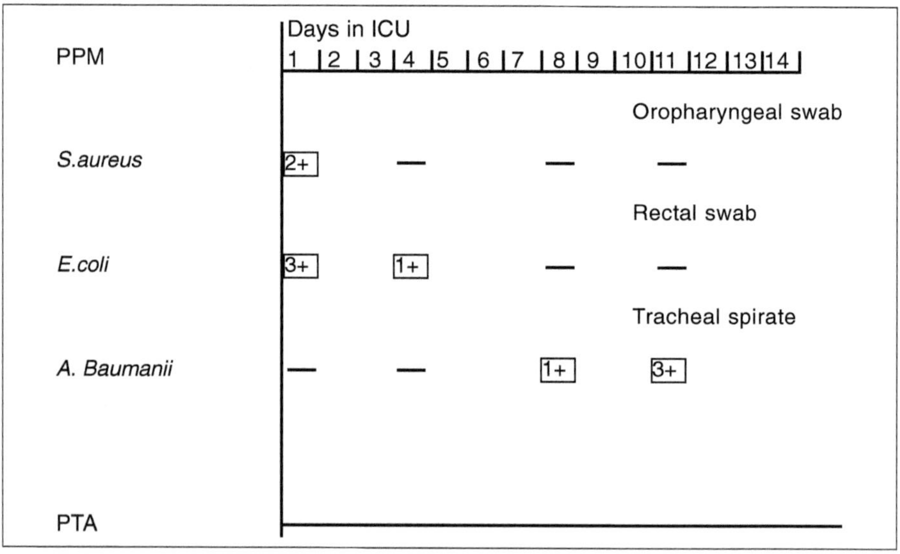

Fig. 2.1 The pathogenesis of an exogenous infection. In an effectively decontaminated patient, i.e. one whose surveillance cultures do not reveal PPM, an *Acinetobacter* species is suddenly isolated from the tracheal aspirate. (PPM, potentially pathogenic microorganism; PTA, polymyxin, tobramycin and amphotericin B)

The major infection problems in the ICU are those caused by primary endogenous infections. Approximately 50% of the infections in the ICU are primary endogenous ones [10, 11]. Primary endogenous infections are caused by PPMs carried in throat and/or gut of the patient on admission (Fig. 2.2). Previously healthy patients such as polytrauma patients or acute liver failure patients, carry only 'community' PPMs in their throat and/or gut besides their low-pathogenetic indigenous flora. During endotracheal intubation these PPMs migrate into the lower airways and, depending on the local and systemic resistance, an infection can develop. Primary endogenous infections can only be prevented by parenteral antimicrobial agents.

The third type of infection, secondary endogenous infection, typically occurs after the first week of ICU treatment (Fig. 2.3). These infections are caused by 'hospital' PPMs, and the major source of these PPM are patients who require long-term intensive care, i.e. other patients-carriers of 'hospital" PPMs. Transmission occurs via the hands of carers. These 'hospital" PPMs are acquired during the first week, and subsequently secondary carriage and overgrowth with PPMs in throat and gut develops, followed by colonisation of the internal organs, such as lower airways and bladder. Depending on the degree of immunoparalysis related to the severity of illness, infection may develop. About 30% of infections in the ICU have a secondary endogenous pathogenesis [10, 11].

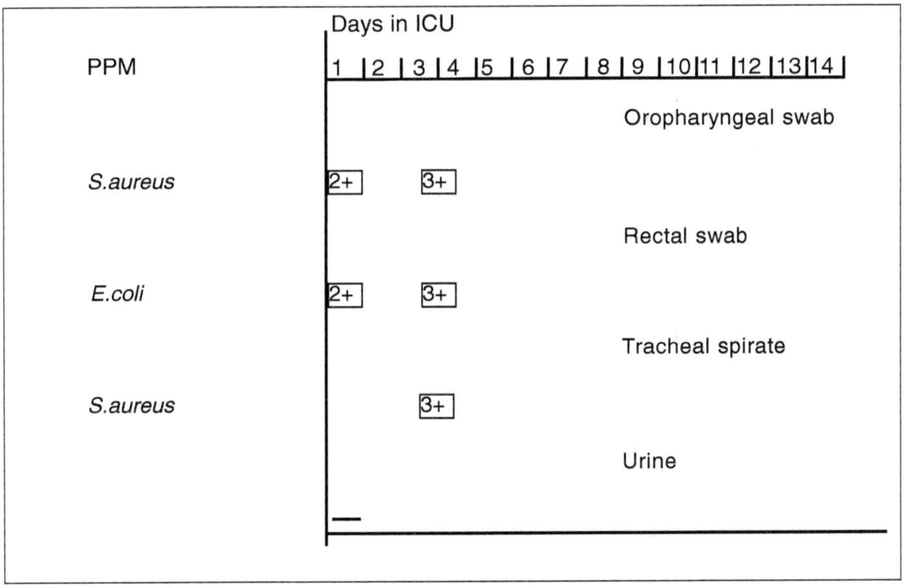

Fig. 2.2 The pathogenesis of a primary endogenous infection. On the 4th day the patient, who was on mechanical ventilation, developed fever and purulent tracheal aspirate, and a new infiltrate seen on the X-ray of the chest. The clinical diagnosis of pneumonia was confirmed by the isolation of +++ *S. aureus* from the tracheal aspirate. *S. aureus* had already been isolated from the surveillance cultures on admission: this pneumonia is a primary endogenous infection

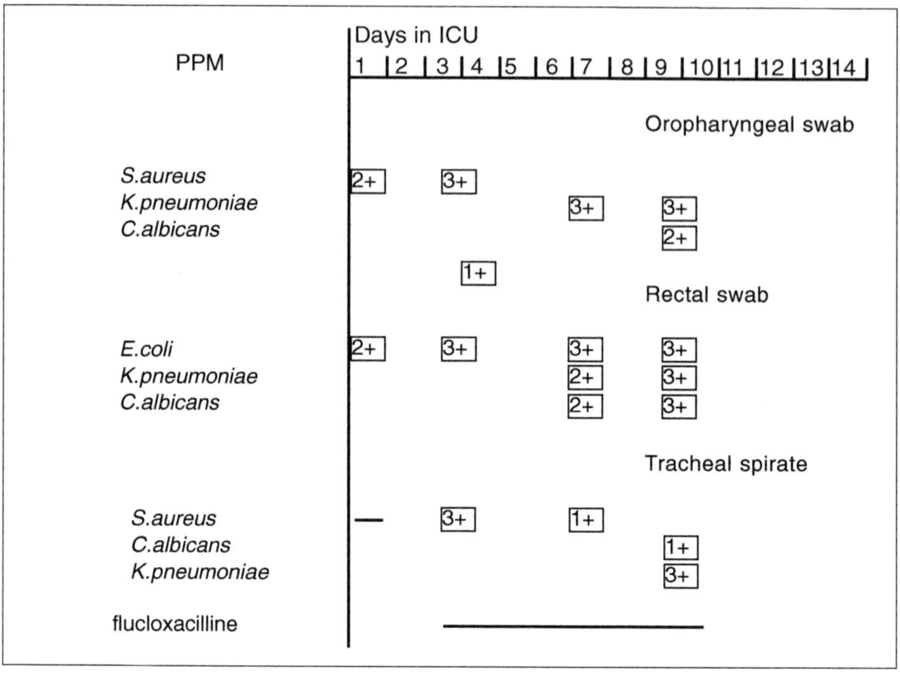

Fig. 2.3 The pathogenesis of a secondary endogenous infection. On the 11th day in the ICU the patient, who was on mechanical ventilation, developped a pneumonia caused by *K. pneumoniae*. This PPM was not isolated from the surveillance cultures obtained on admission to the ICU, indicating that *K. pneumoniae* had been acquired during ICU treatment and carriage in throat and rectum followed. Owing to migration, colonisation and infection of the lower airways occurred: a secondary endogenous infection

The Four-Component Protocol of SDD

The aim of the SDD protocol is to control the three types of infection caused by the 14 (or 15 with MRSA) PPMs. Microorganisms of low virulence, such as enterococci, viridans streptococci, CNS and anaerobes, are left virtually intact, as they do not generally cause serious infections or death. The four elements of the SDD strategy are:

1. A high level of hygiene to prevent exogenous infections. The most important source of PPMs involved in exogenous infections is the long-stay patient who is carrying high concentrations of 'hospital' PPMs in gut and/or throat. These sources can be eradicated using SDD. The inanimate environment is less important as a source of PPMs causing exogenous infections, because the concentrations of PPMs per cm^2 of inanimate devices are low. However, detection and eradication of inanimate sources often require a persistent 'Sherlock Holmes' attitude. Carers, as long as they are healthy, are rarely sources of 'hospital' PPMs.

2. Immediately on admission a parenteral antibiotic is administered to prevent primary endogenous infections. The choice of the antibiotic is important, because recent studies have shown that immediate and adequate antimicrobial therapy reduces mortality in patients admitted to the ICU with an infection [12]. Previously healthy patients with a normal flora can be treated by monotherapy with a beta-lactam antimicrobial. Cefotaxime, a third-generation cephalosporin, is an appropriate choice because it is active against 'community' PPMs. Furthermore, cefotaxime leaves the indigenous, anaerobic flora intact, thus preserving the normal ecology. Patients with a chronic underlying disease, such as alcoholism, poorly regulated diabetes mellitus, or COPD, and patients transferred from other ICUs or general wards are, in general, carrying both 'community' and 'hospital' PPMs in throat and/or gut. Adequate parenteral systemic antibiotic prophylaxis to prevent primary endogenous infection in this group of patients requires combination therapy with an aminoglycoside and cefotaxime until the results of surveillance and diagnostic sampling are reported by the microbiologists. Cefotaxime is replaced by ceftazidime when the patient is suspected of carrying a pseudomonas strain. Parenteral therapy is continued until the end-point of this component of SDD is achieved, or in other words when diagnostic samples taken from the internal organs, such as lower airways and urine, are sterile. Generally this end-point is achieved within 3–5 days.
3. Enteral, nonabsorbable antibiotics, i.e. polymyxin E, tobramycin and amphotericin B (PTA), are applied topically in throat and gut throughout treatment in the ICU to prevent secondary endogenous infections. Four times a day 0.5 g of a sticky paste (Orabase) containing 2% PTA is applied to the oropharyngeal mucosa with a spatula or gloved finger, and 10 ml of a suspension containing 100 mg of polymyxin E, 80 mg of tobramycin and 500 mg of amphotericin B is administered into the gut through a nasogastric tube. All three antimicrobials are nonabsorbable and produce high antimicrobial concentrations of up to 100 times the minimum inhibitory concentrations of the sensitive PPMs in saliva, gastric fluid and faeces. This guarantees eradication of all PPMs from throat and gut. The end-points of this component of the SDD strategy are surveillance samples from throat and rectum that are free of AGNB, yeasts and *S. aureus*.
4. Surveillance cultures from throat and rectum for detection of PPM carriage to distinguish between the three types of infection, to monitor the efficacy of decontamination and to detect the emergence of resistant strains. Surveillance samples are defined as samples from body sites where PPMs are normally carried, i.e. throat, gut and vagina. A set of surveillance samples consists of throat and rectal swabs taken on admission to the ICU and twice weekly thereafter (Monday and Thursday). All data obtained on carriage, colonisation and infection are entered into a database, which can be used to generate a microbiological flowchart for each long-stay patient (Figs. 2.1–2.3). This provides a clear view of trends such as the efficacy of decontamination and allows them to be correlated with other clinical events and treatment.

Traditional Microbiology Versus SDD Microbiology

The crucial difference between the traditional and the SDD approach in critically ill patients is that in the SDD concept surveillance samples from throat and rectum have a central role in the microbiological management of the patient [13]. This routine surveillance of the carrier state of all ICU patients enables the intensive care specialist to monitor the PPMs carried by the patients and the import of new bacteria with every new admission continuously and to distinguish between infections of exogenous and of primary and secondary endogenous pathogenesis. Furthermore, surveillance samples allow the detection of emergence of resistant strains at an early stage and may help to assess the efficacy of PTA, to identify high-risk infection patients and outline empirical antibiotic therapy, assess the level of hygiene in the ICU and control and prevent outbreaks of infection. In contrast, the traditional approach uses diagnostic samples only from normally sterile sites, such as lower airways, bladder and blood. The sole aim of examining these diagnostic samples is to confirm a microbiological cause of inflammation. The second difference is the use of a classification of infections based on the carrier state, while the traditional classification relies on a cut-off time of 48 h to discriminate between community and nosocomial infections. The classification of infections into endogenous, primary and secondary, and exogenous has made it clear that 50% of the infections are primary endogenous ones and are not related to the ICU ecology or breaches of hygiene. It is now evident why the traditional infection prevention measures, such as hand-washing, have failed. The infection control manoeuvres generally recommended cannot be expected to control any but secondary endogenous and exogenous infections.

Conclusion

SDD is a concept requiring commitment from intensivists, nurses and microbiologists. The four-component protocol of SDD consists of a short course of parenteral antimicrobials combined with long-term, enteral, nonabsorbable polymyxin E, tobramycin and amphotericin B, high levels of hygiene and surveillance cultures. The aim is eradication of the target microorganisms, such as AGNB, yeasts and *S. aureus*, resulting in a decline in morbidity and mortality. Effective implementation of the SDD strategy in critically ill patients requires teamwork. Nurses apply the medication and collect the surveillance samples, pharmacists prepare the medication, and the microbiologist processes the samples and reports the results, all under the supervision of the intensivist.

References

1. Baxby D, Van Saene HKF, Stoutenbeek CP et al (1996) Selective decontamination of the digestive tract: 13 years on, what it is and what it is not. Intensive Care Med 22:699-706
2. Silvestri L, Mannucci F, Van Saene HKF (2000) Selective decontamination of the digestive tract: a life saver. J Hosp Infect 45:185-190
3. Rayner BL, Willcox PA (1988) Community-acquired bacteriaemia: a prospective survey of 239 cases. Q J Med 69, 907-919
4. Fagon JY, Chastre J, Domart et al (1989) Nosocomial pneumonia in patients receiving continuous mechanical ventilation. Am Rev Respir Dis 139: 877-844
5. Kerver AJH, Rommes JH, Mevissen-Verhage EAE et al (1987) Colonization and infection in surgical intensive care patient–a prospective study. Intensive Care Med 13:347-251
6. Leonard EM, van Saene HKF, Stoutenbeek CP et al (1990) An intrinsic pathogenicity index for microorganisms causing infection in a neonatal surgical unit. Microbiol Ecol Health Dis 3:151-157
7. Mobbs KJ, van Saene HKF (1999) Oropharyngeal gram-negative bacillary carriage: a survey of 120 healthy individuals. Chest 115:1570-1575
8. Mobbs KJ, van Saene HKF, Sunderland D et al (1999) Oropharyngeal gram-negative bacillary carriage in chronic obstructive pulmonary disease: relation to severity of disease. Respir Med 93:540-545
9. van Saene HKF, Damjanovic V, Murray AE et al (1996) How to classify infections in intensive care units-the carrier state, a criterion whose time has come? J Hosp Infect 33:1-12
10. Silvestri L, Sarginson RE, Hughes J et al (2002) Most nosocomial pneumonias are not due to nosocomial bacteria in ventilated patients. Evaluation of the accuracy of the 48 h time cutoff using carriage as the gold standard. Anaesth Intensive Care 30:275-282
11. Silvestri L, Monti-Bragadin C, Milanese M et al (1999) Are most ICU infections really nosocomial? A prospective observational cohort study in mechanically ventilated patients. J Hosp Infect 42:125-133
12. Alvarez Lerma F and ICU-acquired Pneumonia Group (1996) Modification of empiric antibiotic treatment in patients with pneumonia acquired in the intensive care unit. Intensive Care Med 22:387-394
13. van Saene HKF, Petros AJ, Ramsay G et al (2003) All great truths are iconoclastic: selective decontamination of the digestive tract moves from heresy to level 1 truth. Intensive Care Med 29:677-690

Chapter 3
Infections in Critically Ill Patients: Should We Change to a Decontamination Strategy?

Peter H.J. van der Voort and Hendrick K.F. van Saene

Introduction

Infection in intensive care patients may be the reason for their admission or it may be acquired in the intensive care unit (ICU). Infection in the ICU is common and causes morbidity and hospital mortality [1]. The aim of SDD is to prevent newly acquired infection and associated mortality in the ICU. This chapter describes the magnitude of the infectious problem according to the current literature. If we accept the hypothesis that SDD can prevent ICU acquired infection, it follows that the incidence of infection will show the possible impact of SDD in preventing these infections. However, SDD is designed to prevent infections caused by potentially pathogenic microorganisms (Chapter 2) and will therefore not prevent infections caused by low level pathogens, including coagulase-negative staphylococci and enterococci.

The incidence of infection as the reason for intensive care admission varies according to the type of ICU [2]. For instance, a medical ICU will have a higher prevalence of infection on admission than a cardio-surgical ICU. In the Dutch intensive care database (NICE), 16.1% of patients whose ICU admissions were unplanned had a confirmed infection within 24 h after admission. In the most recent randomised controlled trial (RCT) on SDD, 15–18% of the patients treated with SDD or placebo had an established infection at the time of ICU admission [3]. These primary infections cannot, by definition, be prevented by any infection prevention strategy or antibiotic policy in the ICU. However, it is important to treat these patients with adequate antibiotics as soon as possible [4]. For instance, immediate adequate antibiotic treatment has been shown to improve survival benefit in patients admitted with pneumonia [4, 5].

Secondary or ICU-acquired infections can be prevented by several infection prevention policies. The most important conventional infection prevention policy is hand-washing. Hand-washing can reduce the transmission of potential pathogenic microorganisms but will not eliminate all secondary infections (Chapter 7). This book deals with *Selective Decontamination of the Digestive Tract* as a specific policy designed to prevent secondary infection. In this chapter we will provide an overview of the incidence and prevalence of infections in critically ill patients and explore the possible effects of SDD. In addition to infection prevention, SDD shows the potential to reduce organ failure, especially renal dysfunction [6].

Incidence
The number of new cases of disease occurring in a population during a defined time interval.

Prevalence
The number of individuals with a certain disease in a population at a specified time (point-prevalence) or period of time (period prevalence) divided by the number of individuals in the population at that time.
Note: prevalence does not convey information about risk

Surveys

Infection can be recorded as an incidence in a cohort study (surveillance) or as (point-)prevalence in a cross-sectional study. The surveillance (PREZIES) conducted over 2.5 years in 16 ICUs in The Netherlands showed that 27% of patients treated in ICUs acquired infection in the ICU according to CDC criteria [7]. The most frequent (43%) was pneumonia, followed by sepsis (20%), urinary tract infection (21%) and other infections (16%). The participating ICUs included 12% in which SDD was used, but it was not reported what the infection incidence in these ICUs was relative to those in which SDD was not used.

An example of a point-prevalence study is the European EPIC study [8], which involved 78 ICUs in The Netherlands and 472 patients, 16% of whom had an infection that was acquired in the ICU. Overall, 21% of the patients in the EPIC study had an ICU-acquired infection.

A limited number of other prevalence studies are available on this subject. A French survey over two 3-month episodes showed that the infection rate was 21.6% [9]. VAP was recorded in 9.6% of patients, sinusitis in 1.5%, central venous catheter-associated bacteraemia in 4.8%, catheter-associated urinary tract infection in 7.8% and bacteraemia in 4.5%. The incidence was shown to vary widely between the five participating ICUs. Other surveys have addressed specific patient groups. Papia et al. found in a 1-year survey in hospitalised trauma patients that 37% of them suffered from an infection [10]. In this study 28% of the infections involved the lower respiratory tract, 24% the urinary tract, 18% a wound, and 13% skin/soft tissue; intraabdominal sites accounted for 5% and other sites, for 8%. A survey in a cardiosurgical PICU showed infection rates of 20–25%, decreasing over time [11].

In medical ICUs, the rate of nosocomial infection caused by aerobic gram-negative bacteria (AGNB) was 64%. This rate is the summation of secondary endogenous and exogenous infections. SDD, by preventing gram-negative colonisation, can prevent these infections.

In conclusion, it has been shown that in surveillance studies the incidence of acquired ICU infection affects roughly between 25% and 35% of the patients. Acquired ICU infections can be endogenous or exogenous, a distinction that is not made in the studies mentioned above. The use of surveillance cultures will allow the distinction between primary endogenous and acquired (secondary endogenous or exogenous) infection [12–14]. SDD will be able to reduce endogenous infection but will be less effective in preventing exogenous infection. However, a low colonisation pressure on a ward will decrease the incidence of exogenous infections.

We will discuss the specific infections and the possible role of SDD in the prevention of these infections, dealing with lower airway infections, bloodstream infections, sinusitis, urinary tract infections and wound infections. However, it should be stressed that the clinically important infections on which we should focus in daily clinical care are lower airway infections and bloodstream infections. These are the infections with attributable mortality.

Sites of Infection and the Possible Role of SDD in Prevention

Lower Respiratory Tract Infections

Definition. ICU-acquired pneumonia or ventilator associated pneumonia (VAP) can be defined according to different criteria. The diagnosis is usually made with reference to clinical, radiological and microbiological criteria. In most reviews, studies using different diagnostic strategies and different definitions are all taken together. In one extensive review all aspects, including definition and diagnostic pathways, are discussed [15]. The use of such invasive diagnostic procedures as bronchoalveolar lavage (BAL) or protected specimen brush (PSB) are advised to establish the diagnosis [15]. However, there is no scientific evidence for routine use of these strategies. Fagon et al. demonstrated a reduction in mortality when invasive quantitative versus noninvasive nonquantitative cultures were used to diagnose VAP after 2 weeks, but the significance disappeared after one month [5]. It has recently been shown that endotracheal aspiration and BAL performed for the diagnosis of VAP gave the same results in terms of outcome (mortality) [16].

Epidemiology. Respiratory tract infections are among the most common ICU-acquired infections [17]. In the EPIC point-prevalence study 10% of the patients suffered from pneumonia and 17.8% from tracheobronchitis (for a combined lower airway infection rate of 27%) [8]. However, this point-prevalence study has its limitations. It is far more informative to assess incidence data than prevalence data. For the Dutch situation, the PREZIES study assessed the incidence of pneumonia. It was shown that 43% of the 27% patients who acquired an infection had pneumonia; this was 12% of the ICU population.

Richards reported that the National Nosocomial Surveillance Study revealed that of all nosocomial infections in critically ill medical patients 27% were pneumonia [18]. Eggimann and Pittet, in a review, showed that the incidence of VAP ranged from 6.8% to 35.1% in different studies [19]. The individual RCTs on the effect of SDD on lower airway infection show a wide variation between individual ICUs. The lowest was seen in the study conducted by Jacobs et al., who found 9% in their control group [20], whereas Kerver et al. found an incidence of 85% [21]. The meta-analysis published by d'Amico revealed an overall prevalence of 36% for lower airways infection in the control group for the 30 trials that they included in the analysis [22].

By its nature, SDD is able to prevent secondary endogenous infections (Chapter 2). In addition, the 4-day course of intravenous antibiotics will deal with primary endogenous infections present at the time of ICU admission. Exogenous infections cannot be prevented except by strict hygiene. Thus, to determine the potential effect of SDD on pneumonia we should gain some insight into the nature of respiratory infections. Six studies have now classified respiratory tract infections into primary endogenous, secondary endogenous and exogenous [12–14, 23–25]. Silvestri et al. showed that 60% of the infections in ICU patients were classifiable as primary endogenous and 23% as secondary endogenous [13]. In addition, it was shown that, in burn patients, in 35 of the 37 cases pneumonia was endogenous (21 primary endogenous [57%] and 14 secondary endogenous [38%]) and in two cases was exogenous [23]. For multi-resistant bacteria in a paediatric ICU it was shown that roughly two-thirds of the multi-resistant bacteria were present in the patients on admission (primary and secondary endogenous infections) [12]. True nosocomial infections appear to be the minority, as most patients were carriers of the causal microorganisms at the time of ICU admission [14]. These six studies show that SDD should be able to prevent the secondary endogenous infections, which account for 25–40% of all ICU infections. The systemic antibiotics (usually cefotaxim) that are combined with the SDD suspension will treat the 50–85% primary endogenous infections [12–14, 23–25]. The rate of attributable mortality is 20–30% [26]. The subject of respiratory infection and the effect of SDD on pneumonia incidence and morbidity are discussed in more detail in Chapter 7.

Bloodstream Infections

DiGiovine et al. studied bloodstream infections (BSI) in 3,003 ICU admissions. They found that 68 patients (2.2%) had an ICU-acquired BSI [27]. BSI occurred after median of 10 days in the ICU. Microorganisms involved were coagulase-negative staphylococci (CNS) in 33% of cases, enterococci in 13%, *S. aureus* in 13%, *Candida albicans* in 6% and others (mainly AGNB) in around 34%. The

National Nosocomial Infections Surveillance System (NNIS) found that 19% of all nosocomial infections in medical ICU patients were BSI [18]. There have been 31 studies comparing BSI rates in patients treated with or without SDD. Silvestri et al. recently reviewed them in a meta-analysis [28]. Moreover, a meta-analysis of studies on the effect of SDD on BSI found that the mean incidence of BSI in the control group in the 31 trials analysed was 15%, which was reduced to 11.5% by SDD. Gram-negative BSI was present in 7.1% of the control patients. Gram-positive BSI occurred in 8.2% of the control patients. The design of SDD is appropriate for reduction of Gram-negative BSI insofar as they are endogenous in origin. SDD is by definition not able to prevent CNS-induced and enterococcal BSI. SDD is also not able to prevent exogenous Gram-positive or Gram-negative BSI. Strict hygiene should prevent exogenous infection. However, in a unit with patients on SDD the colonisation pressure with Gram-negatives is low, which should automatically lead to a lower rate than in units where SDD is not used.

The attributable mortality of BSI is lowest for catheter-related BSI (12%); it is 20% for primary bacteraemia and 55% for BSI secondary to nosocomial infection [26].

Sinusitis

The diagnosis of sinusitis may be difficult in ICU patients. Both plain X rays and computed tomography (CT) scans have limited value without bacterial culture of the maxillary sinus secretions [29]. Ultrasound might be an easy bedside technique, but clinical studies in critically ill patients are not available. Radiologically apparent sinusitis may be sterile [30]. In a prospective study the incidence of microbiology-proven (i.e. culture positive) sinusitis in medical ICU patients was 7.7% [31]. Of all nosocomial infections in medical ICU patients, 4% were ear, nose and throat infections, predominantly sinusitis [18]. Van Zanten et al., in a group of critically ill patients with fever of unknown origin, found that 30% were suffering from sinusitis [32]. In 16% of these patients sinusitis was the sole cause of fever, whereas in the other 14% sinusitis was co-existent with some other infection, such as bronchitis. In 101 patients with sinusitis, 140 microorganisms were found, most of them *Pseudomonas* and *Klebsiella* [32]. Sinusitis is usually caused by an overgrowth of pathogenic microorganisms in oral flora that invades the sinus, leading to colonisation and infection. A decreased ability to clear fluids from the sinus by position (supine) and tubes (nasogastric and endotracheal tubes) causes the sinus to become infected. This aetiology suggests that oral decontamination by means of SDD paste will eliminate PPMs from the oral cavity and thus prevent sinusitis. In van Zanten's study, 104 of the 140 different microorganisms found in cultures from sinus drains were potentially susceptible for the SDD medication. Gram-negative microorganisms were found in 65 patients (van Zanten, personal communication). Thus, SDD could have prevented sinusitis in 65 (64%) of the 101 patients. No studies confirming this potential effect of SDD on the prevention of sinusitis are available. On the other hand, our extensive experience with SDD has convinced us that sinusitis is rare in patients receiving SDD and that when it is present it is usually caused by enterococci or coagulase-negative staphylococci. When patients receiving SDD develop fever of unknown origin radiological studies of the sinus should be performed and when there is a suspicion of sinusitis, antral lavage should be performed.

Urinary Tract Infections

The Dutch PREZIES study showed that 21% of the recorded infections in intensive care patients were urinary tract infections (UTI). The EPIC study showed that the point prevalence of UTI was 17.6%. The National Nosocomial Infections Surveillance System in the USA reports that UTI are the most frequently present (31%) nosocomial infections in the ICU [18]; it was observed that 95% of the UTI were associated with indwelling urinary catheters, and half of the patients were symptomatic [18]. Laupland et al. found an incidence of 9% for UTIs in ICU patients who spent more than 48 h in the ICU [33]. *Enterococcus* species were found in 24% of the patients, and *Candida* species in 21%. Rosser et al. made a retrospective study of the incidence of ICU-acquired urosepsis [34]. They found that of 126 patients with ICU-acquired sepsis, 15.8% (20 patients) had urosepsis. They showed low specificity for both urinalysis and urine culture, but the combination could be used to make the diagnosis. Independent risk factors were: age >60 years, extended length of stay in the ICU and relatively long duration of urinary catheterisation. The causative microorganisms were *Pseudomonas, Staphylococcus, Escherichia coli* and *Acinetobacter* species. For 10% of the UTIs the microorganisms involved were not shown. However, at least 80% of UTI are due to aerobic Gram-negative bacteria (AGNB), which can be prevented by SDD. Similarly, Paradisi et al., in a review, observe that AGNB are the most prevalent microorganisms [35]. Indeed, two RCTs show a significant reduction in UTI in patients receiving SDD [6, 36]. Krueger found a reduction in urinary tract infection from 22.9% to 13.6% (36 vs 60 patients, p=0.045) [6]. Rocha found a reduction in urinary tract infections from 31% in the control group to 9% in the decontaminated group (p = 0.01) [36].

Apparently, these were secondary endogenous infections by origin, which have been shown to be preventable by the use of SDD.

Wound Infections

SDD, by definition, can prevent secondary endogenous wound infections caused by AGNB, *S. aureus* and yeasts. The topical antibiotics, PTA, cover these target microorganisms. *S. aureus*, which is usually involved in wound infection, is adequately treated with cefotaxime. A significant effect of SDD on the prevention of wound infections was established by the results of the original SDD study by Stoutenbeek [37]. It was shown that wound infection decreased from 25% to 5% in SDD-treated trauma patients. In burn patients a correlation was found between colonisation of the gastrointestinal tract and wound colonisation [38]. This specific patient group is described further in Chapter 14.

Impact of SDD on Infections Classified Into Gram-Negative and Gram-Positive and Yeast Infections

Two meta-analyses assessing the impact of SDD on Gram-negative, Gram-positive and yeast infections are available [39, 40]. The first meta-analysis of 54 RCTs involved a total of 9,473 patients, and the primary end-points were Gram-negative and Gram-positive infections [39]. There were 42 RCTs with a total of 6,075 critically ill patients in the second meta-analysis, which had fungal infections as the primary end-point [40].

Infections Attributable to AGNB

The rate of infection attributable to AGNB was 18.8% in the controls and 4.4% in patients receiving SDD [39]. SDD significantly reduced AGNB infections by 83% (OR 0.17, 95% CI 0.10–0.28, $p<0.001$). Six patients needed to be treated to prevent one infection with AGNB (NNT 6.93, 95% CI 6.89–6.97). Lower airway infections due to AGNB developed in 3.2% and 22.7%, respectively, of the patients with SDD and without SDD. The SDD prophylaxis significantly reduced the odds ratio (OR) of AGNB lower airway infections (OR 0.11, 95% CI 0.06–0.2, $p<0.01$). Five patients needed to be treated with SDD to prevent one lower airway infection with AGNB (NNT 5.12, 95% CI 5.09–5.16).

The prevalence of AGNB BSI was 7.7% amongst controls and 2% amongst patients receiving SDD [28]. Eighteen patients needed to be treated with SDD to prevent one BSI with AGNB (NNT 17.76, 95% CI 17.74–17.79).

Infections Attributable to Gram-Positive Bacteria

The infection rate in the control group was 10.3%, whilst in the patients receiving SDD the rate was 9.4% [39]. SDD reduced overall infections due to Gram-positive bacteria, albeit not significantly (OR 0.76, 0.41–1.40). However, lower airway infections were significantly reduced (OR 0.52; 95% CI 0.34–0.78, p = 0.0016), whilst Gram-positive BSI were not significantly increased by SDD (OR 1.03, 95% CI 0.75–1.41, p = 0.85) [28].

Fungal Infections

It is generally accepted that the incidence of secondary (nosocomial) fungal infections in the ICU has increased over the years [17], from 2 to 3.8 nosocomial fungal infections per 1,000 discharges over the period 1980–1990 in the USA, for example [41]. Its incidence at all organ sites rose in this period, particularly that of BSI. Patients in the ICU are particularly prone to fungal infections because of major surgery, burns, indwelling vascular catheters, parenteral nutrition, assisted ventilation and haemodialysis [42]. In addition, most ICU patients have received extensive antibiotic therapy leading to widespread yeast carriage and overgrowth. Yeast carriage has been shown to be an independent risk factor for fungal infection. It has been shown that increasing colonisation enhances the risk of infection [23].

The aim of SDD is the eradication and prevention of secondary colonisation of PPM, including AGNB and yeast. When carriage and overgrowth promote infection, it is assumed that reducing carriage will lead to a decrease in fungal infections. Indeed, carriage of yeasts was decreased with an odds ratio of 0.32, and fungal infections under SDD were reduced with an odds ratio of 0.30 [40]. Surprisingly, the incidence of fungaemia was not reduced by SDD.

There were 20 patients with fungal infections in the SDD group (20/1,577, 1.3%) and 62 in the control group (62/1,605, 3.9%). These data demonstrate that SDD significantly reduces the incidence of fungal infection (OR 0.30, 95% CI 0.17–0.55). Thirty-eight patients needed to receive SDD to prevent one fungal infection (NNT 38.54, 95% CI 38.53–38.55) [40].

Clostridium Difficile

Specific infection with *Clostridium difficile* occurs in patients pretreated with antimicrobials that disregard their intestinal ecology. In particular, ICU patients who are treated i.v. with antibiotics are at risk of developing *Clostridium difficile* infection. SDD implies that antibiotics are routinely administered. However, *Clostridium difficile* infection is extremely uncommon [43] (D.F. Zandstra, personal communication; authors' own experience). The mechanism behind the protective effect of SDD is respect for normal indigenous flora providing colonisation resistance by anaerobes and Gram-positive bacteria (mainly enterococci). The colonisation resistance prevents *Clostridium difficile* from being acquired and from colonising the digestive tract. It is of the utmost importance for patients treated with SDD that intravenous antibiotics that respect colonisation resistance be selected (Chapter 15). In practice, this implies a very restricted use of penicillin-like antimicrobials, as enterococci and anaerobes are susceptible to this class of antibiotics. One RCT comparing patients with and without SDD carefully screened for *Clostridium difficile* toxins in all patients with diarrhoea and was unable to detect this toxin in the stool samples [43].

Conclusion

It has been shown that around 30% of ICU patients acquire infection whilst being treated in the ICU. Lower airway infection and BSI are by far the most important clinically. Most of these infections are preventable by nature, as they are secondary endogenous infections. It is shown that the vast majority of AGNB-related respiratory infections, BSI and urinary tract infections are preventable. In addition, sinusitis and yeast infections can also be prevented by the application of SDD.

References

1. Osmon S, Warren D, Seiler SM et al (2003) The influence of infection on hospital mortality for patients requiring >48 h of intensive care. Chest 124:1021-1029
2. Wenzel RP, Thompson RL, Landry SM et al (1983) Hospital acquired infection in intensive care unit patients: An overview with an emphasis on epidemics. Infect Control 4:371-375
3. De Jonge E, Schultz M, Spanjaart L et al (2003) Selective decontamination of the digestive tract. Lancet 362:1011-1016
4. Alvarez-Lerma F (1996) Modification of empiric antibiotic treatment in patients with pneumonia acquired in the intensive care unit. ICU-Acquired Pneumonia Study Group. Intensive Care Med 22:387-394
5. Fagon JY, Chastre J, Wolff M et al (2000) Invasive and non-invasive strategies for management of suspected ventilator-associated pneumonia. A randomised trial. Ann Intern Med 132:621-630
6. Krueger WA, Lenhart FP, Neeser G et al (2002) Influence of combined intravenous and topical antibiotic prophylaxis on the incidence of infections, organ dysfunctions, and mortality in critically ill surgical patients: a prospective, stratified, randomized, double-blind, placebo-controlled clinical trial. Am J Respir Crit Care Med 166:1029-1037
7. Mintjes-de Groot AJ, Geubbels ELPE, Beaumont MTA et al (2001) Ziekenhuisinfecties en risicofactoren op de intensive-care afdelingen van 16 Nederlandse ziekenhuizen; resultaten van surveillance als indicator voor zorgkwaliteit. Ned Tijdschr Geneesk 145:1249-1254
8. Vincent JL, Bihari DJ, Suter PM et al (1995) The prevalence of nosocomial infection in intensive care units in Europe (EPIC) JAMA 274(8):639-644
9. Legras A, Malvy D, Quinioux AI et al (1998) Nosocoomial infections: prospective survey of incidence in five French intensive care units. Intensive Care Med 24:1040-1046
10. Papia G, McLellan BA, El-Helou P et al (1999) Infection in hospitalised trauma patients: incidence, risk factors, and complications. J Trauma 47:923-927
11. Dagan O, Cox PN, Ford-Jones L et al (1999) Nosocomial infection following cardiovascular surgery. Comparison of two periods, 1987 vs. 1992. Crit Care Med 27:104-108
12. Petros AJ, O'Connel M, Roberts C et al (2001) Systemic antibiotics fail to clear multidrug-resistant Klebsiella from a pediatric ICU. Chest 119:862 866
13. Silvestri L, Monti Bragadin C, Milanese M et al (1999) Are most ICU infections really nosocomial? A prospective observational cohort study in mechanically ventilated patients. J Hosp Infect 42:125-133
14. Silvestri L, Sarginson RE, Hughes J et al (2002) Most nosocomial pneumonias are not caused by nosocomial bacteria in ventilated patients. Evaluation of the accuracy of the 48 hours time cut-off as the gold standard. Anaesth Intensive Care 30:275-282
15. Chastre J, Fagon JY (2002) Ventilator associated pneumonia. Am J Respir Crit Care Med 165:867-903

16. Heyland D, Dodek P, Muscedere J et al (2006) A randomized trial of diagnostic techniques for ventilator-associated pneumonia. N Engl J Med 355:2619-2630
17. Wallace WC, Cinat ME, Nastanski F et al (2000) New epidemiology for postoperative nosocomial infections. Am Surg 66:874-878
18. Richards MJ, Edwards JR, Culver DH et al (1999) Nosocomial infections in medical intensive care units in the United States. National Nosocomial Infections Surveillance System. Crit Care Med 27:887-892
19. Eggimann P, Pittet D (2001) Infection control in the ICU. Chest 120:2059-2093
20. Jacobs S, Foweraker JE, Roberts SE (1992) Effectiveness of selective decontamination of the digestive tract in an ICU with a policy encouraging a low gastric pH. Clin Intensive Care 3:52-58
21. Kerver AJ, Rommes JH, Mevissen-Verhage EA et al (1988) Prevention of colonization and infection in critically ill patients: a prospective randomized study. Crit Care Med 16:1087-1093
22. D'Amico R, Pifferi S, Leonetti C et al (1998) Effectiveness of antibiotic prophylaxis in critically ill adult patients: systematic review of randomized controlled trials. BMJ 316:1275-1285
23. De la Cal MA, Cerda E, Garcia-Hierro P et al (2001) Pneumonia in patients with severe burns. A classification according to the concept of the carrier state. Chest 119:1160-1165
24. Murray AE, Chambers JJ, van Saene HKF (1998) Infections in patients requiring ventilation in intensive care: application of a new classification. Clin Microbiol Infect 4:94-99
25. Sarginson RE, Taylor N, Reilly N et al (2004) Infection in prolonged pediatric critical illness: a prospective four-year study based on knowledge of the carrier state. Crit Care Med 32:839-847
26. Marshall JC, Marshall KAM (2005) ICU-acquired infection: mortality, morbidity, and costs. In: van Saene HKF, Silvestri L, de la Cal MA (eds) Infection control in the intensive care unit, 2nd edn. Springer-Verlag, Milan, pp 605-620
27. DiGiovine B, Chenoweth C, Watts C et al (1999) The attributable mortality and costs of primary nosocomial bloodstream infections in the intensive care unit. Am J Respir Crit Care Med 160:976-981
28. Silvestri L, van Saene HKF, Milanese M et al (2007) Selective decontamination of the digestive tract reduces bacterial bloodstream infection: and mortality in critically ill patients. Systematic review of randomized, controlled trials. J Hosp Infect 65:187-203
29. Skoulas IG, Helidonis E, Kountakis SE (2003) Evaluation of sinusitis in the intensive care unit patient. Otolaryngol Head Neck Surg 128:503-509
30. Rouby JJ, Laurent P, Gosnach M et al (1994) Risk factors and clinical relevance of nosocomial maxillary sinusitis in the critically ill. Am J Respir Crit Care Med 150:776-783
31. George DL, Falk PS, Meduri GU et al (1998) Nosocomial sinusitis in patients in a medical intensive care unit: a prospective epidemiological study. Clin Infect Dis 27:463-470
32. Van Zanten ARH, Dixon JM, Nipshagen MD et al (2005) Hospital-acquired sinusitis is a common cause of fever of unknown origin in orotracheally intubated critically ill patients. Crit Care 9:R583-590
33. Laupland KB, Zygun DA, Davies HD et al (2002) Incidence and risk factors for acquiring nosocomial urinary tract infection in the critically ill. J Crit Care 17:50-57
34. Rosser CJ, Bare RL, Meredith JW (1999) Urinary tract infections in the critically ill patient with a urinary catheter. Am J Surg 177:287-290
35. Paradisi F, Corti G, Mangani V (1998) Urosepsis in the critical care unit. Crit Care Clin 14:165-180
36. Rocha LA, Martin MJ, Pita S et al (1992) Prevention of nosocomial infection in critically ill patients by selective decontamination of the digestive tract. A randomised, double blind, placebo-controlled study. Intensive Care Med 18:398-404
37. Stoutenbeek CP, van Saene HK, Miranda DR et al (1984) The prevention of superinfection in multiple trauma patients. J Antimicrob Chemother 14 Suppl B: 203-211

38. Manson WL, Klasen HJ, Sauer EW et al (1992) Selective intestinal decontamination for prevention of wound colonization in severely burned patients: a retrospective analysis. Burns 18:98-102
39. Silvestri L, van Saene HKF, Casarin A et al (2007) Reducing the carrier state controls severe infections in the critically ill; systematic review of 54 randomised controlled trials of selective decontamination of the digestive tract. Chest (submitted for publication)
40. Silvestri L, van Saene HKF, Milanese M et al (2005) Impact of selective decontamination of the digestive tract on fungal carriage and infection: systematic review of randomized controlled trials. Intensive Care Med 31:898-910
41. Beck-Sague CM, Jarvis WR, and the National Nosocomial Infections Surveillance System (1993) Secular trends in the epidemiology of nosocomial fungal infections in the United States, 1980-1990. J Infect Dis 167:1247-1251
42. Rogers TH (1998) Nosocomial fungal infections in intensive care unit patients. In: van Saene HKF, Silvestri L, de la Cal MA (eds) Infection control in the intensive care unit. Springer-Verlag 1998, Milan, pp 144-151
43. Cockerill FR 3rd, Muller SR, Anhalt JP et al (1992) Prevention of infection in critically ill patients by selective decontamination of the digestive tract. Ann Intern Med 117:545-553

Chapter 4
Gut Microbiology: How to Use Surveillance Samples for the Detection of the Carrier Status of Abnormal Flora

Hendrick K.F. van Saene

Introduction

Critical illness impacts on all organ systems, such as lungs, heart and gut. This last organ also includes the vast living microbial tissue of the indigenous, mainly anaerobic, flora. That enormous bacterial tissue is embedded in the mucous layer and covers the inner wall of the gut. Of all aerobic Gram-negative bacilli (AGNB), the indigenous *Escherichia coli* is the only one carried in the gut by healthy people . It is critical illness that converts the status of normal carriage of *E. coli* into carriage of abnormal AGNB, including *Klebsiella, Enterobacter, Pseudomonas* species and methicillin-resistant *Staphylococcus aureus* (MRSA) [1]. It is hypothesised that receptors for AGNB and MRSA are constitutively expressed on the mucosal lining, but are covered by a protective layer of fibronectin in the healthy mucosa. Significantly increased levels of salivary elastase have been shown to precede AGNB carriage in the oropharynx in postoperative patients and in the elderly [2, 3]. It is probable that in individuals suffering both acute and chronic underlying illness, activated macrophages release elastase into mucosal secretions, thereby denuding the protective fibronectin layer. It is thought that this possible mechanism is a deleterious consequence of the inflammatory response encountered during and after illness. This shift towards abnormal flora as a result of underlying disease is aggravated by most iatrogenic interventions in the septic patient. Gut protection using H_2 antagonists raises gastric pH, thereby impairing the gastric acidity barrier [4]. Antimicrobials that are active against the indigenous, mainly anaerobic, flora and are excreted via bile into the gut may disturb the gut ecology [5]. Both factors—integrity of the physiology and of the flora—are essential for the individual's defence against carriage of AGNB. Impairment of these two factors promotes the overgrowth of abnormal potentially pathogenic microorganisms (PPM) such as AGNB in concentrations of more than 10^5 colony-forming units (CFU) per millilitre (ml) or gram (g) of faeces [6].

Gut overgrowth of abnormal flora is not only a marker of critical illness; this particular condition harms the patient, being a disease in itself. In addition, gut overgrowth of abnormal flora has a major epidemiological impact on the other patients in the ICU and in the ICU environment.

Acquisition
The act or process of acquiring a microorganism in the gut.

Carrier status/carriage
The presence of a microorganism in two or more surveillance samples.

Overgrowth
The presence of more than 10^5 identical microorganisms in a microbiological sample.

Colonisation
The populating of new areas by a species; or: the presence of a microorganism in one sample from a normally sterile site.
Note: in the USA colonisation is also used for the gut.

Infection
A microbiological proven local or systemic inflammation. The diagnostic sample yields at least 10^5 bacteria.

Clinical Impact of Gut Overgrowth

Intestinal overgrowth with AGNB causes systemic immunoparalysis [7]. Together with the depressed immunity, high concentrations of AGNB and MRSA in throat and gut may result into pneumonia [8] and septicaemia [9] following aspiration into the lower airways and translocation in the terminal ileum. Amongst the AGNB population gut overgrowth guarantees the presence of antibiotic-resistant strains producing enzymes that neutralise the antimicrobials [10]. The salivary and faecal concentrations of the parenterally administered antimicrobials are generally not bactericidal for the PPM present in high numbers in the gut, and they create an environment in which antibiotic-resistant strains readily survive.

There is an epidemiological impact of gut overgrowth: the higher the salivary and faecal concentrations of AGNB and MRSA, the higher the likelihood of PPM transmission via the hands of carers [11–13]. Acquisition of PPM invariably leads to carriage, as the critically ill are unable to clear the acquired AGNB and MRSA. Carriers of abnormal bacteria in overgrowth shed these microorganisms into the environment and determine the contamination level of the inanimate environment, including beds, tables, telephones and floor [14].

Definitions

Surveillance samples are defined as samples obtained from body sites where PPM may potentially be carried, e.g. the digestive tract comprising of the oropharyngeal and rectal cavities [15]. Surveillance cultures must be distinguished from surface and diagnostic samples. *Surface samples* are taken from the skin, e.g. in the axilla, groin and umbilicus, and from the nose, eye and ear. They do not belong in a surveillance sampling protocol, because positive surface swabs merely reflect the oropharyngeal and rectal carrier states. *Diagnostic samples* are samples from internal organs that are normally sterile, such as lower airways, blood, bladder and skin lesions. They are only taken on clinical indication. The end-point of diagnostic samples is clinical, as they aim to provide microbiological confirmation of a clinical diagnosis of inflammation, both generalised and/or local.

End-points

The aim of obtaining surveillance cultures is to determine the microbiological end-point of the carrier status for potentially pathogenic microorganisms [16]. Carriage or a carrier status exists when the same bacterial strain is isolated from at least two consecutive surveillance samples of the ICU patient in any concentration over a period of at least one week. Carriage implies persistent presence of a PPM, and a distinction is made between it and acquisition or transient presence. Surveillance samples are not useful for diagnosing infection of lungs, blood, bladder or wounds, diagnostic samples are required for this purpose.

Sampling for surveillance purposes

What patients? Only in the subset of the most critically ill patients is intensive microbiological monitoring using surveillance samples required for detection of the abnormal carriage of AGNB and MRSA. Owing to the severity of their illness these patients need intensive care including mechanical ventilation for at least three days. They generally have impaired gut motility and are therefore at high risk of developing throat and gut overgrowth.

What samples? A surveillance programme for patients of this type includes samples from both oropharynx and gut. Potential pathogens carried in throat and gut cause pneumonia [8] and septicaemia [9], respectively. These two serious infections are responsible for mortality. Potential pathogens present in overgrowth in throat and gut are implicated in transmission via the hands of carers, especially in outbreak situations. A throat and a rectal swab are taken to detect the oropharyngeal and gut carriage of AGNB and MRSA. Rectal swabs are required to be coated with stool. As MRSA has an affinity for the skin, skin is sampled only if lesions are present.

When? Surveillance sets are obtained on admission and thereafter twice weekly (e.g. on Mondays and Thursdays) throughout the ICU stay, in order to distinguish carriage due to PPM imported in the admission flora ("import") from carriage caused by ICU-associated PPM acquired in the oropharynx and gut during the ICU stay ("nosocomial", "secondary" or "super" carriage).

Microbiological procedures

Throat and rectal swabs are processed qualitatively and semi-quantitatively, including an enrichment broth, to detect the level of carriage of the three types of target microorganisms, AGNB, *S. aureus* sensitive and resistant to methicillin, and yeasts [1, 16-17].

Three solid media, MacConkey (AGNB), staphylococcal, and yeast agar, are inoculated using the four-quadrant method, and a brain–heart infusion broth culture designed to detect low-grade carriage is included (Fig. 4.1). Each swab is streaked onto the three solid media, and then the tip is broken off into 5 ml of enrichment broth. All cultures are incubated aerobically at 37°C. The MacConkey plate is examined after one night and the plates for staphylococci and yeasts, after two nights. In addition, if the enrichment broth is turbid after a one-night incubation, it is then inoculated onto the three media. A semi-quantitative estimation is made by grading growth density on a scale of 1+ to 5+, as

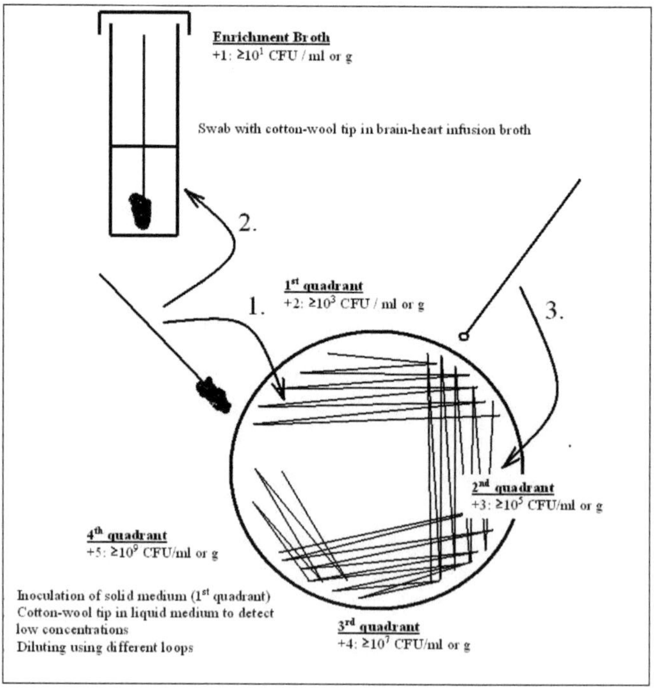

Fig. 4.1 Processing surveillance swabs using the four-quadrant method and enrichment step: *1* Inoculation of solid medium (1st quadrant); *2* Cottonwool tip in liquid medium to detect low concentration; *3* Diluting using different loops

follows (Table 4.1): growth in broth only = 1+ (approx. 10 microorganisms/ml), growth in the first quadrant of the solid plate = 2+ (≥10^3 CFU/ml), in the second quadrant = 3+ (≥10^5 CFU/ml), in the third quadrant = 4+ (≥10^7 CFU/ml), and on the whole plate = 5+ (≥10^9 CFU/ml). Macroscopically distinct colonies are isolated in pure culture. Standard methods for identification, typing and sensitivity patterns are used for all microorganisms. All data are entered in the computer. A simple programme enables the intensive care specialist to view the microbiological overview chart of each long-stay patient at the bedside. Figures 4.2 and 4.3 show typical examples.

Table 4.1 Comparison of the surveillance (throat/rectal) swabs and (salivary/faecal) specimens for the detection of the level (growth density) of carriage of aerobic brown-negative bacilli, *Staphylococcus aureus* both sensitive and resistant to methicillin, and yeasts

Four-quadrant method with enrichment step Semi-quantitative swab method	Growth density	Dilution series Quantitative specimen method
1+	Very low	10^1
2+	Low	10^3
3+	Moderate	10^5
4+	High	10^7
5+	Very high	10^9

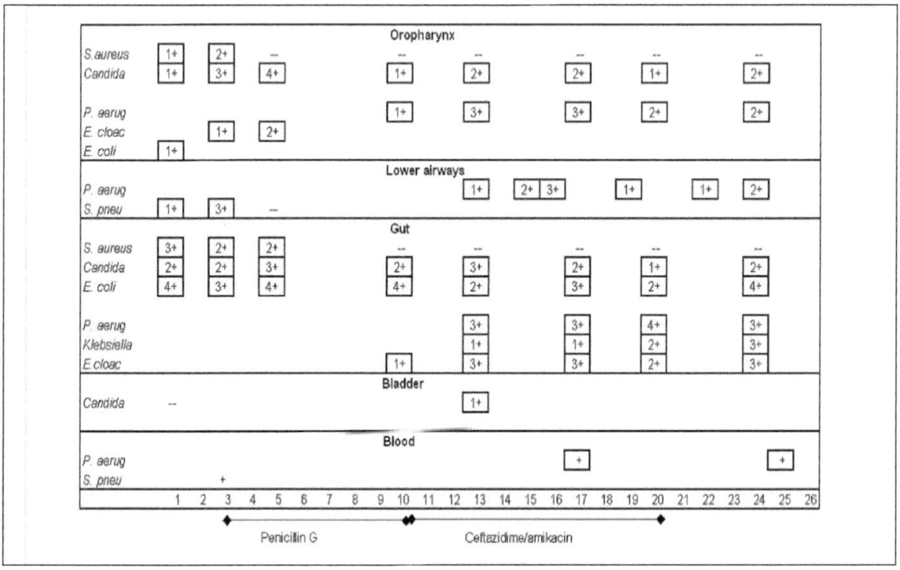

Fig. 4.2 Oropharyngeal and gastrointestinal carriage detected by surveillance samples shown in combination with the colonisation/infection data obtained in the diagnostic samples from lower airways, bladder and blood. The overview chart shows that both primary and secondary endogenous infections occur after 48 hours

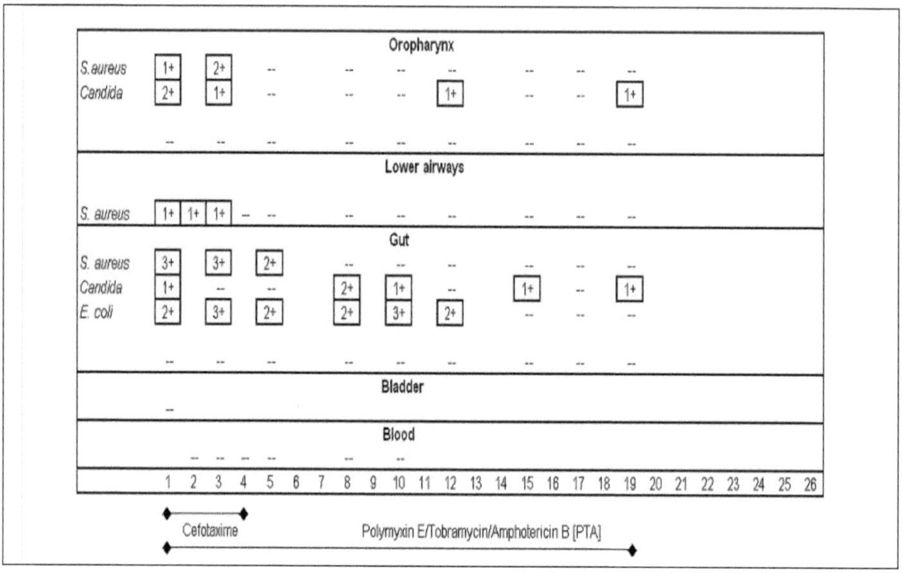

Fig. 4.3 This microbiological chart shows the pattern of a trauma patient who received the full protocol of selective decontamination of the digestive tract (SDD) immediately on admission. Cefotaxime controlled primary endogenous infection developing within the first week, and topical polymyxin E/tobramycin/amphotericin B [PTA] prevented the development of super-carriage and subsequent supercolonisation and infection

Interpretation of Surveillance Samples

Surveillance cultures allow the intensive care specialist to distinguish the normal from the abnormal carrier status, overgrowth from low-level carriage, and endogenous from exogenous infections when examined in combination with diagnostic samples.

Normal vs abnormal carriage. Surveillance swabs processed for one group of target microorganisms, AGNB, using an inexpensive MacConkey agar plate yield a positive or negative result after 18 h of incubation. AGNB including *E. coli* are uncommon in the oropharynx, whilst healthy people carry their own indigenous *E. coli* in the intestine in concentrations varying between 10^3 and 10^6 CFU per ml or g of faeces [17] (Table 4.2). There are no other AGNB, including *Klebsiella, Proteus, Morganella, Enterobacter, Citrobacter, Serratia, Acinetobacter,* and *Pseudomonas* species, in either throat or gut. Before interpretation of the staphylococcal plate is possible two nights of incubation are required. About one third of the healthy population carries methicillin-sensitive *S. aureus*. The isolation of methicillin-resistant *S. aureus* or MRSA is always abnormal [1]. Yeasts also require 48 hours of incubation, and they can be carried by approximately 30% of the healthy adult population in concentrations of <3+ or <10^5 CFU per ml of saliva and per g of faeces. However, yeast overgrowth promotes translocation and fungaemia.

Table 4.2 Surveillance cultures: normal and abnormal values

Source	Normal values	Abnormal values
1. Throat	*S. aureus*/*C. albicans* (30% carriage)	*S. aureus*/*C. albicans* (30% carriage)
Swab	<3+ CFU/ml	≥3+ CFU/ml
Saliva	$<10^5$ CFU/ml	$>10^5$ CFU/ml *E. coli*, AGNB, MRSA in any concentration
2. Rectum	Indigenous *E. coli* (100% carriage) *S. aureus* / *C. albicans* (30% carriage)	Indigenous *E. coli* (100% carriage) *S. aureus* / *C. albicans* (30% carriage)
Swab	<3+ CFU/g	≥3+ CFU / g
Faeces	$<10^5$ CFU/g	$\geq 10^5$ CFU /g AGNB / MRSA in any concentration
3. Vagina	See rectum	See rectum

Low-grade carriage vs overgrowth. Oropharyngeal and intestinal overgrowth is defined as ≥3+ or $\geq 10^5$ micro-organisms per ml of saliva and/or g of faeces and is distinguished from low-grade carriage of <3+ or $<10^5$ micro-organisms [1, 6, 17]. Individuals with a chronic disease such as chronic obstructive pulmonary disease carry abnormal flora, generally in low concentrations, once the forced expiratory volume in 1s is <50% [18]. The low-level carrier status is mainly due to the presence of clearing mechanisms such as swallowing, chewing and peristalsis. However, patients who require mechanical ventilation for minimally three days generally have impaired gut motility and readily develop overgrowth [19]. Gut overgrowth has been shown to be an independent risk factor for (1) colonisation/infection of internal organs [8, 9], (2) the expression of an antibiotic-resistant mutant among the microbial population [10], and (3) transmission of (often antibiotic-resistant) microorganisms [11–13].

'Imported' versus 'nosocomial' carriage. Knowledge of the carrier status, at admission and subsequently, is crucial to the management of infection on the ICU. Hygiene measures will only have an impact on infections caused by externally transmitted microorganisms. A primary endogenous infection caused by a PPM imported into the ICU by the patient in the admission flora can only be managed effectively when the carrier state is known. It is obvious that hand hygiene fails to eradicate carriage in throat and gut detected by surveillance samples on admission. However, that information enables the intensivist to implement isolation and to reinforce hygiene measures as soon as possible following admission. Two recent studies show that MRSA and ceftazidime-resistant AGNB were identified in 23.8% and 52.1% of the patients within the first 72 hours of admission to the ICU [20, 21].

Interaction between carriage and infection. With the structured approach, which combines data from surveillance and diagnostic samples (Figs. 4.2, 4.3, Table 4.3), infection can be categorized into three different groups [22]:

Table 4.3 Strengths and weaknesses of both surveillance methods: infection only and infection combined with carriage

Strengths	Weaknesses
Surveillance of infection (solely diagnostic samples)	*Surveillance of infection (solely diagnostic samples)*
Already routine	Cost effectiveness: has to be tested
Not controversial	Time cut off of 48h: not accurate for the estimation of infections due to ICU microorganisms
Number of infections per 1000 device days: of value within one unit	Value of this method for interhospital comparison: limited Detection of resistant micro-organisms, of transmission, impending outbreak, exogenous problem: always late
Surveillance of infection and carriage (diagnostic samples combined with surveillance samples)	*Surveillance of infection and carriage (diagnostic samples combined with (surveillance samples)*
More accurate estimation of infections due to ICU-associated microorganisms	Workload for laboratory is higher
Early identification of exogenous problem	Surveillance samples are unpopular amongst traditional microbiologists
Early detection of resistant microorganisms	Cost effectiveness has to be tested
Detection of transmission at an early stage	Value of method for interhospital comparison: has to be tested
Indispensable in control of an outbreak	

a. Primary endogenous infections are the most frequent; their incidence varies between 60% and 85% depending on the severity of illness of the patient population studied [23–26]. They are caused by both "community" and "hospital" microorganisms carried in the throat and gut on admission. These episodes typically occur within the first week in the ICU. Examples include lower airway infection in a previously healthy individual caused by *Streptococcus pneumoniae*, or "hospital"-type organisms such as *Klebsiella pneumoniae* in patients with underlying disease. Adequate parenteral antibiotics, e.g. cefotaxime given immediately on admission and for 4 days, will reduce the incidence of primary endogenous infection [27–29].

b. Secondary endogenous infections are caused by ICU-associated microorganisms appearing late in the patient's stay in the ICU, in general after one week [23]. These ICU microorganisms are first acquired in the oropharynx, followed by the stomach and gut. One third of ICU infections are secondary endogenous infections [23–26]. Significantly, of patients who are antibiotic free on admission, almost only those who have previously had a primary endogenous infection develop a secondary endogenous infection; that is to say there is a subset of critically ill patients who develop more than one infection during their stay in the ICU [25]. Only the topical application of nonabsorbable antimicrobials polymyxin E/tobramycin/amphotericin B (PTA) throughout the stay in the ICU has been shown to control secondary endogenous infection [11–13].
c. Exogenous infections are less common (approximately 15%) [23–26], but can occur throughout the patient's stay on ICU and are caused by "hospital" bacteria, in particular *Acinetobacter* spp., *Pseudomonas* spp. and MRSA without previous carriage. Typical examples are lower airway infections caused by *Acinetobacter* spp. in patients with a tracheostomy, whether or not they receive PTA [30, 31]. A high level of hygiene is required to control exogenous infections [32].

To control the three types of infection that can occur in the ICU, enteral PTA antimicrobials are added to the parenteral cefotaxime, whilst a high level of hygiene is maintained all the time. Surveillance samples from throat and rectum are an integral part of this infection control program for the septic patient, for the following reasons: (1) to monitor the compliance and efficacy of PTA; (2) to detect any exogenous problem in the ICU; and (3) to detect the emergence of resistant microorganisms at an early stage. SDD is the full four-component strategy (SDD) [33–35].

Role of Surveillance Samples in Infection Control in the Septic Patient

Recent studies using surveillance cultures of throat and rectum to detect the carrier state demonstrate that only infections occurring after one week of the patient's stay in the ICU are due to microbes transmitted via the hands of health-care workers [23–26]. The incidence varies between 15% and 40%, depending on the severity of illness. Microorganisms related to the ICU environment are first acquired in the oropharynx. In the critically ill, oropharyngeal acquisition invariably leads to secondary or super-carriage. The subsequent build-up to digestive tract overgrowth, which can then result in colonisation of normally sterile internal organs, takes a few days. Finally, it is the degree of immune suppression of the ICU patients that determines the day of colonisation leading to an established *secondary endogenous* or superinfection. The other type of ICU infection is the *exogenous* infection attributable to breaches of hygiene [30–32]. The causative bacteria are also acquired on the unit but are never present in the throat and/or gut flora of patients. For example, long-stay patients, particularly those who undergo tracheostomy in respiratory units, are at high risk of exogenous lower airway infections. Purulent lower airway secretions yield a microorganism that has never previously been carried by these patients in their digestive tract flora, or indeed in their oropharynx. Although both the tracheostomy and the oropharynx are equally accessible for bacterial entry, the tracheostomy tends to be the entry site for bacteria, which colonise/infect the lower airways. However, the major infection problem is *primary endogenous* infection, and the microorganisms involved do not bear any relation to the ecology of the ICU. A recent study compared the traditional 48-hours cut-off and the criterion of the carrier status to find that the time cut-off significantly overestimated the magnitude of the nosocomial problem [26]. This approach to knowledge of the carrier status may be more useful for interhospital comparison, as only infections that are due to microorganisms acquired in the different units are compared, regardless of the severity of illness.

With regard to infection control for the septic patient (Table 4.3), by identifying the right population with primary endogenous infections, the classification by carrier status avoids blaming staff for all infections after 48 hours for which they are not responsible. Knowledge of the carrier status thus prevents fruitless investigation of apparent cross-infection episodes. Secondly, without surveillance samples it is not possible to recognise exogenous infections, at least at an early stage when only diagnostic samples, such as tracheal aspirate, urine and blood, have been tested. Finally, knowledge of the carrier status derived from surveillance cultures taken on admission and twice weekly thereafter is an effective strategy for the early identification of carriers of multi-resistant microorganisms including AGNB, such as *Acinetobacter baumannii* [36], MRSA [21, 23, 37] and vancomycin-resistant enterococci [38], both on admission and during the stay in the ICU. When surveillance cultures, in particular from the oropharynx, become positive for a PPM during a patient's stay in the ICU, this reveals ongoing transmission and an impending outbreak long before the diagnostic samples yield the outbreak strain [39]. This surveillance strategy optimises targeted infection control interventions, including (1) hand hygiene; (2) isolation; (3) personal protective equipment; and (4) care of the patient's equipment to control transmission from one patient-carrier to another via the hands of carers.

Future Lines of Research on Surveillance Samples in the Septic Patient

Most infection surveillance programmes include all patients admitted to the ICU whether they stay a few days or 2 weeks [40, 41]. The inclusion of a large number of relatively short-stay patients with a low risk of infection tends to dilute the total rates of infection by increasing the size of the denominator. However, low percentages look good to hospital managers but do not allow room for improvement as they obscure detection of any significant reduction in infection rate following the introduction of an intervention [24]. We believe that septic patients benefit from a programme of surveillance of both infection and carriage [42], in particular in combination with SDD [33–35].

Acknowledgements. We are very grateful to Mrs Lynda Jones for her meticulous typing of the manuscript and to Drs Derrick Baxby, Luciano Silvestri and Miguel-Angel de la Cal for careful review.

References

1. van Saene HKF, Damjanovic V, Alcock SR (2001) Basics in microbiology for the patient requiring intensive care. Curr Anaesth Crit Care12:6-17
2. Dal Nogare AR, Toews GB, Pierce AK (1987) Increased salivary elastase precedes Gram-negative bacillary colonization in postoperative patients. Am Rev Respir Dis 135:671-675
3. Palmer LB, Albulak K, Fields S et al (2001) Oral clearance and pathological oropharyngeal colonisation in the elderly. Am J Respir Crit Care Med 164:464-468
4. Hillman KM, Riordan T, O'Farrell SM et al (1982) Colonization of the gastric contents in critically ill patients. Crit Care Med 10:444-447
5. Vollaard EJ, Clasener HAL (1994) Colonization resistance. Antimicrob Agents Chemother 38:409-414
6. Husebye E (1995) Gastro-intestinal motility disorders and bacterial overgrowth. J Intern Med 237:419-427
7. Marshall JC, Christou NV, Meakins JL (1988) Small-bowel bacterial overgrowth and systemic immuno-suppression in experimental peritonitis. Surgery 104:404-411
8. van Uffelen R, van Saene HKF, Fidler V et al (1984) Oropharyngeal flora as a source of bacteria colonizing the lower airways in patients on artificial ventilation. Intensive Care Med 10:233-237
9. Luiten EJT, Hop WCJ, Endtz HP et al (1998) Prognostic importance of gram-negative intestinal colonization preceding pancreatic infection in severe acute pancreatitis. Intensive Care Med 24:438-445
10. Damjanovic V, Van Saene HKF (2005) Microbial mutation as a source of polyclonality in the gut of the critically ill. J Hosp Infect 59:374-375
11. Tayler ME, Oppenheim BA (1991) Selective decontamination of the digestive tract as an infection control measure. J Hosp Infect 71:271-278
12. Damjanovic V, Connolly CM, van Saene HKF et al (1993) Selective decontamination with nystatin for control of a Candida outbreak in a neonatal intensive care unit. J Hosp Infect 24:245-259
13. Silvestri L, Milanese M, Oblach L et al (2002) Enteral vancomycin to control methicillin-resistant Staphylococcus aureus outbreak in mechanically ventilated patients. Am J Infect Control 30:391-399
14. Go ES, Urban C, Burns J et al (1994) Clinical and molecular epidemiology of Acinetobacter infections sensitive only to polymyxin B and sulbactam. Lancet 344:1329-1332
15. Damjanovic V, van Saene HKF, Weindling AM (1994) The multiple value of surveillance cultures: an alternative view. J Hosp Infect 28:71-78
16. Mobbs KJ, van Saene HKF, Sunderland D et al (1999) Oropharyngeal Gram-negative bacil-

lary carriage. A survey of 120 healthy individuals. Chest 115:1570-1575
17. Crossley K, Solliday J (1980) Comparison of rectal swabs and stool cultures for the detection of gastro-intestinal carriage of Staphylococcus aureus. J Clin Microbiol 11:433-434
18. Mobbs KJ, van Saene HKF, Sunderland D et al (1999) Oropharyngeal Gram-negative bacillary carriage in chronic obstructive pulmonary disease: relation to severity of disease. Respir Med 93:540-545
19. van der Spoel JI, Oudemans-van Straaten HM, Stoutenbeek CP et al (2001) Neostigmine resolves critical illness-related colonic ileus in intensive care patients with multiple organ failure – a prospective, double-blind, placebo-controlled trial. Intensive Care Med 27:822-827
20. Toltzis P, Yamashita T, Vilt L et al (1997) Colonization with antibiotic-resistant Gram-negative organisms in a pediatric intensive care unit. Crit Care Med 25:538-544
21. Viviani M, van Saene HKF, Dezzoni R et al (2005) Control of imported and acquired methicillin-resistant Staphylococcus aureus (MRSA) in mechanically ventilated patients: a dose-response study of enteral vancomycin to reduce absolute carriage and infection. Anaesth Intensive Care 33:361-372
22. van Saene HKF, Damjanovic V, Murray AE et al (1996) How to classify infections in intensive care units – the carrier state, a criterion whose time has come? J Hosp Infect 33:1-12
23. Silvestri L, Monti Bragadin C, Milanese M et al (1999) Are most ICU-infections really nosocomial? A prospective observational cohort study in mechanically ventilated patients. J Hosp Infect 42:125-133
24. Petros AJ, O'Connell M, Roberts C et al (2001) Systemic antibiotics fail to clear multi-drug-resistant Klebsiella from a pediatric ICU. Chest 119:862-866
25. de la Cal MA, Cerda E, Garcia-Hierro P et al (2001) Pneumonia in patients with severe burns. A classification according to the concept of the carrier state. Chest 119:1160-1165
26. Silvestri L, Sarginson RE, Hughes J et al (2002) Most nosocomial pneumonias are not due to nosocomial bacteria in ventilated patients. Evaluation of the 48h time cut-off using carriage as the gold standard. Anaesth Intensive Care 30:275-282
27. Stoutenbeek CP (1989) The role of systemic antibiotic prophylaxis in infection prevention in intensive care by SDD. Infection 17:418-421
28. Sirvent JM, Torres A, El-Ebiary M et al (1997) Protective effect of intravenously administered cefuroxime against nosocomial pneumonia in patients with structural coma. Am J Respir Crit Care Med 155:1729-1734
29. Alvarez-Lerma F, and the ICU-pneumonia study group (1996) Modification of empiric antibiotic treatment in patients with pneumonia acquired in the intensive care unit. Intensive Care Med 22:387-394
30. Hammond JMJ, Potgieter PD, Saunders GL et al (1992) Double blind study of selective decontamination of the digestive tract in intensive care. Lancet 340:5-9
31. Morar P, Singh V, Makura Z et al (2002) Differing pathways of lower airway colonization and infection according to mode of ventilation (endotracheal versus tracheotomy). Arch Otolaryngol Head Neck Surgery 128:1061-1066
32. Morar P, Makura Z, Jones AS et al (2000) Topical antibiotics on tracheostoma prevents exogenous colonization and infection of lower airways in children. Chest 117:513-518
33. Baxby D, van Saene HKF, Stoutenbeek CP et al (1996) Selective decontamination of the digestive tract: 13 years on, what it is and what it is not. Intensive Care Med 22:699-706
34. D'Amico R, Pifferi S, Leonetti C et al (1998) Effectiveness of antibiotic prophylaxis in critically ill adult patients: systematic review of randomized controlled trials. BMJ 316:1275-1285
35. Nathens AB, Marshall JC (1999) Selective decontamination of the digestive tract in surgical patients. A systematic review of the evidence. Arch Surg 134:170-176
36. Corbella X, Pujol M, Ayats J et al (1996) Relevance of digestive tract colonization in the epidemiology of nosocomial infections due to multiresistant Acinetobacter baumannii. Clin Infect Dis 23:329-334

37. de la Cal MA, Cerda E, van Saene HKF et al (2004) Effectiveness and safety of oral vancomycin to control endemicity of methicillin-resistant Staphylococcus aureus in a medical/surgical intensive care unit. J Hosp Infect 56:175-183
38. Hendrix CW, Hammond JMJ, Swoboda SM et al (2001) Surveillance strategies and impact of vancomycin-resistant enterococcal colonization and infection in critically ill patients. Ann Surg 233:259-265
39. Silvestri L, Petros AJ, Sarginson RE et al (2005) Handwashing in the intensive care unit: a big measure with modest effects. J Hosp Infect 59:172-179
40. Kollef MH, Sherman G, Ward S et al (1999) Inadequate antimicrobial treatment of infections. Chest 115:462-474
41. Richards MJ, Edwards JR, Culver DH et al (1999) Nosocomial infections in medical intensive care units in the United States. Crit Care Med 27:887-892
42. Langer M, Carretto E, Haeusler EA (2001) Infection control in ICU: back (forward) to surveillance samples? Intensive Care Med 27:1561-1563

Chapter 5
Compounding Medication for Digestive Decontamination: Pharmaceutical Aspects

Rients Schootstra and Jan P. Yska

Introduction

To assess the effect of selective decontamination of the digestive tract on respiratory tract infections and survival of patients treated in an intensive care unit, meta-analyses of clinical studies comparing patients treated with selective decontamination and untreated controls have been carried out. Analyses of these studies have shown a protective effect of selective decontamination on infections. On the other hand, the mortality benefit has been shown only recently [1]. Earlier studies with historical controls and randomised trials showed that mortality was not significantly different between treatment and control patients. The evidence from these studies is consistent with an effect of selective decontamination of the digestive tract on survival of patients in the intensive care unit, in addition to a clear preventive effect on the occurrence of respiratory tract infections [2–12].

Owing to the lack of any lowering of mortality that could supply convincing evidence supporting the concept of selective decontamination in previous studies, doctors and other medical professionals tend to be either "believers" or "nonbelievers" in selective decontamination. In the discussions between these two groups pharmaceutical aspects hardly ever play a crucial role. However, the new evidence may lead to increased use of SDD. For selective decontamination of the digestive tract a standardised combination of amphotericin B, colistin sulphate (polymyxin E) and tobramycin sulphate is used in the forms of mouth paste, suspension and suppository. However, in the case of MRSA, vancomycin administered as a mouth paste and via a nasogastric tube as a solution may be considered [13–16]. In this chapter, we will try to emphasise the importance of pharmaceutical aspects of the standardised combination. We find these so important that we believe the effect of selective decontamination will stand or fall with the input of adequate pharmaceutical knowledge and effort. We are breaking a lance for a more prominent role of pharmacists in the design and performance of clinical trials on selective decontamination. The pharmacist is a crucial factor in proper application of SDD, as the products required for it are not readily avail-

P.H.J. van der Voort, H.K.F. van Saene (eds.) *Selective Digestive Tract Decontamination in Intensive Care Medicine*. © Springer 2008

able from the shelf. The pharmaceutical industry does not produce a commercially available product. The local pharmacist must manufacture the topical agents.

Pharmacotherapy in a hospital is a complex healthcare technology. In most countries, nurses generally prepare and administer drugs prescribed by doctors. Administration of drugs has been associated with considerable risk [17]. In several countries drug errors have become prime targets in increasing patient safety [18, 19]. Little prospective research has been done into the incidence, causes and severity of drug errors. Single-site studies have been carried out and have indicated error rates of 13–84% in preparation and administration of drugs [20–23], but such studies used different definitions and did not assess the severity of errors. When this is borne in mind, it is easy to imagine that the performance of selective decontamination according to a pharmacotherapeutic protocol on a ward or in an intensive care unit involves a certain risk in itself [24, 25].

The essence of this risk is quite simple; it can even be expressed in an arithmetic formula as the product of a usually negative outcome and probability. This makes it possible to balance between poor and unsatisfactory outcome on the one hand and better and more satisfactory outcome on the other. This knowledge can be used in outcome calculations and outcome assessments, but finding a way to determine probabilities in an objective, unbiased, and thus correct, way may pose a problem. From a pharmaceutical point of view, one way of improving a system, i.e. all procedures concerning selective decontamination, is to describe the entire process analytically and try to obtain quantitative data on the failure rate of every step in the process. This might allow identification of the most critical parts of the chain and, in turn, more effective improvement of the entire process. In fact, in a highly complex system such as the process of selective decontamination of the digestive tract, there are so many chances of an unsatisfactory outcome that the analysis of all possible causes probably reflects imagination rather than reality. In other words, it is not hard to imagine where things would go wrong [26]. Risk assessment in this field is a powerful tool to improve unbiased outcome in a proactive manner. It needs systematic trend analysis and a good understanding of all steps in the process of selective decontamination of the digestive tract (SDD).

The Special Nature of Drugs Used in SDD

Drugs are special insofar as they generally have a great potential for good but, if wrongly prepared or wrongly administered, may cause much harm. Yet, no other products are taken so totally on trust: "Nothing of so great importance to human welfare is used more completely on faith than a medicinal product" [27]. The consumer of drugs, i.e. the patient (or his/her nurse and/or doctor), takes a drug entirely on trust in the vast majority of cases. There is no way of knowing whether it contains active substances, whether it is the right substance, whether the dosage prescribed is correct, or whether any contaminants or degradation products are present. The ultimate consumer, the patient in the ICU, is almost never in a position to recognise when a drug is incorrect or defective. He or she is at one end of a chain of implicit trust, which extends back through administering, dispensing, prescribing and distributing, right back to the hospital pharmacist who is responsible for manufacturing the product. All along the line there is an implicit trust that the pharmacist has done his job properly. The social and moral implications of this "chain of trust" alone are sufficient to make medicines, and their manufacture and quality assurance, "special". Another factor that makes drugs "special" is the problem of testing them. There are very great potential hazards if even only small quantities of defective ingredients are present within one batch, and yet these might well remain undetected by anything less than 100% testing. Furthermore, it has been shown impossible to test a drug for everything that might be "wrong" about it, in terms of formulation error, mix-up, contamination or degradation. Still another special factor is the profound effect that formulation changes and changes in the method of processing may have on the safety and efficacy of the end-product.

Therefore, it can be quite clearly stated that the approach to quality assuring of the drugs to be used in selective decontamination needs to be especially rigorous.

Quality as "Fitness for Purpose"

When compounding a drug formulation a pharmacist must manufacture this formulation so as to ensure that it is fit for its intended use. Furthermore, it should not place the patient at risk by inadequate safety, quality or efficacy.

For all this to be achieved, the process of designing, compounding and quality control has to be part of a larger quality management system. In the pharmaceutical industry quality management has been legally anchored in legislation on the safety of medicines and in good manufacturing practice (GMP). In hospital pharmacy a quality system should be implemented that is based on the GMP guidelines so far as the compounding of medicinal products is concerned. The Pharmaceutical Inspection Convention (PIC/S) is developing a guide to good practices for preparation of medicinal products in pharmacies.

Quality management involves all activities within a hospital that are aimed at achieving quality. The quality system reflects the organisation of quality management. Quality control involves operational techniques and activities used to fulfil quality requirements. In order to be able to ensure the supply of SDD products of good quality, both the compounding department and the pharmaceutical laboratory of the pharmacy perform such 'operational techniques and activities'. This part of quality control, which concerns measuring and testing, is also included in Quality Control in the GMP guidelines. Quality control, however, apart from the performance of final examinations, also requires involvement in in-process controls and in validation and drafting of compounding procedures and methods of preparation. Quality assurance introduces and monitors all planned and systematic activities within this quality system.

The pillars of modern quality management are the presence of a quality system consisting of the following parts:

- An organisational structure with clearly defined tasks, responsibilities and qualifications;
- A well-structured and sufficiently detailed documentation system;
- Personnel who have sufficient knowledge of quality management and are highly motivated to achieve good quality;
- Availability of the necessary facilities and resources;
- Audits.

Two Major Aspects of Quality

All efforts to manufacture medicines for SDD will be wasted if there is any flaw or omission in their original design that renders them fundamentally unfit or inadequate. It is thus conventional and proper quality theory to distinguish between two separate, but interrelated, aspects of quality:

- Quality of design;
- Quality of compounding.

Quality of Design

The quality of the design of the formulation and the compounding instructions for medicinal products, i.e. SDD formulations, that are prepared in the pharmacy do not have to be licensed. However, formulations should have an appropriate quality of design. Since it concerns nonlicensed medicinal products, quality has not been established by way of licensing.

In the hospital pharmacy distinction can be made between standardised and nonstandardised preparations. Standardised preparations are preparations that are manufactured in the pharmacy on a regular basis, as stock preparations or by extemporaneous compounding, and for which sufficient guarantees are available for it to be possible to guarantee the quality. Guidelines for this purpose are summarized in Table 5.1.

Quality of compounding

The design of the compounding starts with the assessment of the pharmacotherapeutic purpose and the rationale behind it. Next, the pharmaceutical quality has to be optimised. With due consideration for both the basic principles of SDD and the

Table 5.1 Guidelines for quality of design of formulation and instructions for preparation

1	The design of the formulation and the preparation instruction should be laid down in a procedure. The assessment of the pharmacotherapeutic rationality and safety should be included in this procedure.
2	In the case of limited availability of data on the quality of design, the risks for the patient resulting from this lack of information should be weighed against the risks of not supplying the requested preparation.
3	A documentation file should be made for each preparation.
4	Biopharmaceutical and pharmaceutical-technical aspects should be considered in the design of the formulation.
5	In designing the formulation and the preparation instruction it is permissible to use data obtained from the literature and data yielded by investigations performed by others.
6	Specifications for active ingredients, other starting materials and primary packaging materials should be determined on the basis of legal and professional requirements.
7	Stability of the preparations should be well founded.
8	In the instructions for preparation the method of preparation should be described step by step. This description should include all critical steps and the corresponding in-process controls.
9	Sampling and the way in which the final examination has to be performed should be laid down.
10	Standardised preparation instructions should be validated before their use in stock preparation.
11	Validation should be repeated if there has been an essential change in formulation, materials, method of preparation or equipment.
12	Formulation and preparation instruction should be authorised, at least by the pharmacist who bears the responsibility for the preparation.

biopharmaceutical characteristics, for SDD procedures the oropharyngeal, oral and rectal routes have been determined as the necessary routes of administration.

Furthermore, attention must be paid to the feasibility of applying the preparation with regard to the available facilities, its chemical and physical stability, the method of preparation, patient requirements, determination of starting materials and auxiliary substances, and patient information, for example.

A batch compounding instruction contains a list of the active ingredients and other starting materials to be used, the equipment and the utensils to be used, and a stepwise description of the operations to be performed in chronological order. For the monitoring of the critical points in the preparation, in-process controls are included.

Which compounding steps will actually be the critical points in a preparation depends on the nature of the SDD preparation in question, but also on batch size, used equipment and personnel. In-process controls per dosage form have to be set up.

At a minimum, the following data should be documented before and/or during the preparation:

- Source of the method
- Quantity to be delivered
- Batch size
- Active ingredients and other starting materials
- Packaging materials to be used
- Protective measures for personnel
- Instructions on the preparation
- In-process controls
- Starting materials used and weighed quantities
- Quality control results
- Authorisation of the design
- Release signature

The Active Substances

For a hospital pharmacy, it is of crucial importance that active pharmaceutical ingredients are purchased from manufacturers who follow the European guidelines for GMP and who have a quality management system in place to guarantee the necessary quality. The manufacturer of active substances for SDD should have implemented the current GMP guidelines on active pharmaceutical ingredients from the European Agency for the Evaluation of Medicinal Products (ICH Q 7 A). In a hospital pharmacy, the analysis of incoming materials from a qualified manufacturer of active ingredients may be limited. Containers should be undamaged and have a clear label. The active substances to be used in the compounding of drugs for SDD, amphotericin B, tobramycin sulphate and colistin sulphate (polymyxin E), should meet the requirements of the European Pharmacopoeia or The United States one. The substances should always be sent together with a specification and certificate of analysis. For an example of a certificate of analysis from a qualified supplier see Table 5.2. For positive identification, infrared spectroscopy may be used. Further testing of additional parameters in pharmacopoeia monographs is not required.

Amphotericin B is a mixture of antifungal polyenes and is a yellow or orange powder that is practically insoluble in water. It is sensitive to light in dilute solutions and is inactivated at low pH values. Amphotericin B, suitable for use in the manufacture of parenteral dosage forms, should be sterile and free from bacterial endotoxins and contain 5% or less amphotericin A, a tetraene which is less active than amphotericin B. However, for the manufacture of drugs for oral or

Table 5.2 Example of a Certificate of Analysis of Amphotericin B from a qualified supplier (note)

FÄHRHAUS Pharma

Bramfelder Strasse 123a – D-22305 Hamburg – Tel. +49- 40 / 61 17 18 19 – www.faehrhaus-pharma.de

Certificate of Analysis

Substance: Amphotericin B

Batchnumber: **FP03086A** Manufacturing date: **February 2003**
CAS-No: **1397-89-3** Retest date: **January 2005**

Parameter	Specification PH.EUR. 2002	Results
Assay with reference to the dried substance [a]As it is	min. 750 I.U. / mg	948 I.U. / mg 906 I.U. / mg
Description	Yellow or orange powder	Complies
Solubility	Practically insoluble in water, soluble in dimethyl sulfphoxide and in propylene glycol, slightly soluble in dimethylformamide, very slightly soluble in methanol, practically insoluble in ethanol	Complies
Identification: UV spectrum IR absorption spectrum Colour in solution	Maxima at 362, 381 and 405 nm. Comparison with reference spectrum. Blue and yellow colour is produced	Complies Complies Complies
Content of tetraenes	max. 10,0% (Parenteral dosage forms max. 5,0%)	4,89%
Loss on drying	max. 5,0%	4,57%
Sulphated ash	max. 3,0%	0,14%
Aerobic microbial counts	max. 1000 c.f.u. / g	530 c.f.u. /g
Residual solvents	Methanol max. 3000 ppm Acetone max. 5000 ppm	329 ppm 111 ppm
STORAGE: PROTECTED FROM LIGHT AND AT A TEMPERATURE OF 2-8¡C!		
The substance corresponds to the PH.EUR. 2002 specification		

Note: FÄHRHAUS Pharma is now Fagron

topical use the amphotericin B should contain 10% or less amphotericin A; it is not necessary for the substance to be sterile and free from bacterial endotoxins. More detailed information is listed in Tables 5.3 and 5.4 and in Fig. 5.1.

Table 5.3 Amphotericin B: chemical properties

CAS no.	1397-89-3
EINECS no.	215-742-2
Chemical formula	$C_{47}H_{73}NO_{17}$
Molecular weight	924.08

Table 5.4 Pharmacopoeial description of amphotericin B

European Pharmacopoeia	A mixture of antifungal polyenes produced by the growth of certain strains of *Streptomyces nodosus* or by any other means. It consists largely of amphotericin B. It occurs as a yellow or orange powder. The potency is not less than 750 units per mg with reference to the dried substance. It contains not more than 10% of tetraenes, or not more than 5% if intended for use in parenteral dosage forms. Practically insoluble in water and in alcohol; soluble in dimethyl sulfoxide and in propylene glycol; slightly soluble in dimethyl formamide; very slightly soluble in methyl alcohol. Amphotericin B is sensitive to light in dilute solutions and is inactivated at low pH values.
USP 29	A yellow to orange, odorless or practically odorless, powder. It contains not less than 750 micrograms of $C_{47}H_{73}NO_{17}$ per mg, and, for material intended for oral or topical use, not more than 15% of amphotericin A, both calculated on the dried substance. Insoluble in water, in dehydrated alcohol, in ether, in benzene, and in toluene; soluble in dimethylformamide, in dimethylsulfoxide, and in propyleneglycol; slightly soluble in methylalcohol. Store at a temperature not exceeding 8 degrees in airtight containers. Protect from light.

Tobramycin sulphate is an aminoglycoside antibiotic with good aqueous solubility. It is effective against many strains of Gram-negative bacteria, including *Pseudomonas aeruginosa*. More detailed information is listed in Tables 5.5 and 5.6 and in Fig. 5.2.

Colistin is a multicomponent antibiotic. It consists of a mixture of several closely related decapeptides (polymyxin E). As many as 13 components have been identified. The main components are polymyxin E1 and E2. Colistin has an antimicrobial spectrum and mode of action similar to that of polymyxin B, but

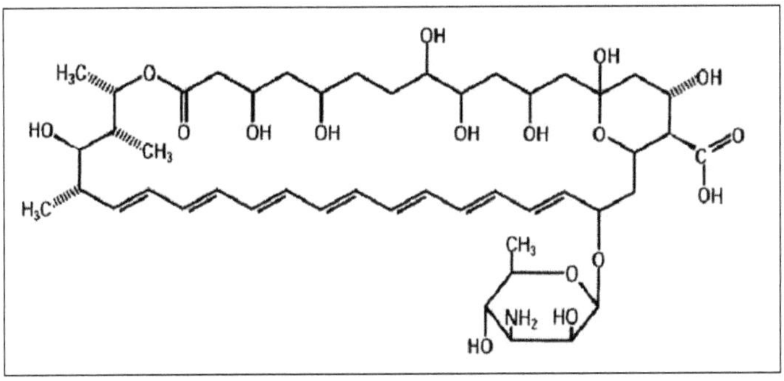

Fig. 5.1 Structural formula of amphotericin B

Table 5.5 Tobramycin sulphate: chemical properties

CAS no.	79645-27-5
EINECS no.	256-499-2
Chemical formula	$C_{18}H_{37}N_5O_9\ H_2SO_4$
Molecular weight	467.52

Table 5.6 Pharmacopoeial description of tobramycin sulphate

USP 29	Tobramycin sulfate has a potency of not less than 634 micrograms and not more than 739 micrograms of tobramycin per mg. A 4% solution in water has a pH of 6.0 to 8.0. Store in airtight containers.

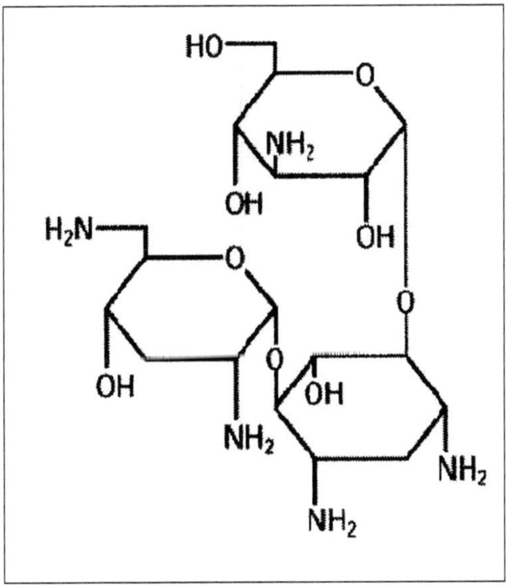

Fig. 5.2 Structural formula of tobramycin sulphate

it is slightly less active. It has a bactericidal action on most Gram-negative bacteria. As the sulphate colistin is a white or almost white powder, freely soluble in water. Its physicochemical characteristics are as follows:

- The base is precipitated from aqueous solution above pH 7.5.
- The first International Standard Preparation (1968) for colistin contains 20,500 units per milligram of colistin sulphate.

More detailed information on colistin sulphate is shown in Tables 5.7 and 5.8 and in Fig. 5.3.

Table 5.7 Colistin sulphate: chemical properties

CAS no.	1264-72-8
EINECS no.	215-034-3
Chemical formula	$C_{45}H_{85}N_{13}O_{10}$ H_2SO_4
Chemical name	Mixture of colistin A, B and C; polymyxin E
Molecular weight	1169.47

Table 5.8 Pharmacopoeial description of colistin sulphate

European Pharmacopoeia	A mixture of the sulphates of polypeptides produced by certain strains of *Bacillus polymyxa* var. colistinus or obtained by any other means. The potency is not less than 19 000 units per mg, calculated with reference to the dried substance. A white or almost white, hygroscopic powder. Freely soluble in water; slightly soluble in alcohol; practically insoluble in acetone and in ether. A 1% solution in water has a pH of 4.0 to 6.0. Store in airtight containers. Protect from light.
USP 29	The sulfate salt of an antibacterial substance produced by the growth of *Bacillus polymyxa* var. colistinus. It has a potency of not less than 500 micrograms of colistin per mg. A white to slightly yellow, odorless, fine powder. Freely soluble in water; insoluble in acetone and in ether; slightly soluble in methyl alcohol. pH of a 1% solution in water is between 4.0 and 7.0. Store in airtight containers.

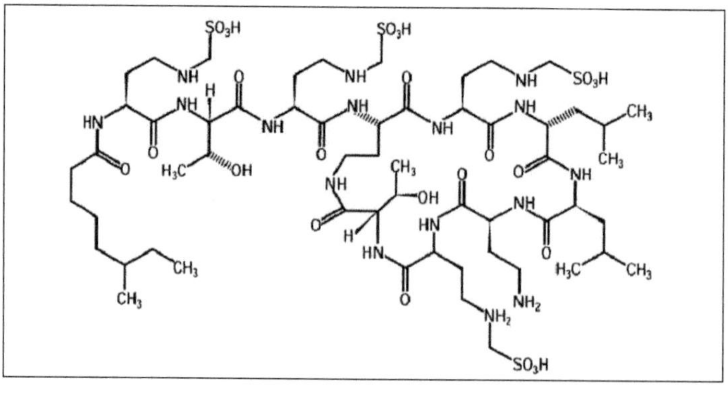

Fig. 5.3 Structural formula of colistin sulphate

Dosage Forms of Drugs for SDD

As the oropharyngeal, the oral and rectal routes of administration have been selected for medicines used for SDD, formulations had to be designed that would be fit for this purpose. Hence, an oral paste, a suppository and an oral suspension have been developed (Figs. 5.4-5.6).

a. SDD oral paste 15 g

Ingredients:

Saccharoid sodium	100 mg
Tobramycin sulphate	462 mg
Colistin sulphate	303 mg
Amphotericin B	303 mg
Methylhydroxypropylcellulose 4000 mPa.s	2,500 mg
Menthae piperitae aetheroleum	61 μl
Paraffin liquidum 110–230 mPa.s	3,939 mg
Vaselinum album	7,800 mg

Packaging material:
Collapsable metal tube (see Fig. 5.4).

The oral paste contains:

Amphotericin B	2%
Colistin sulphate	2%
Tobramycin (as sulphate)	2%

Storage temperature: between 4 °C and 8 °C
Stability: 6 months

b. SDD suspension for gastroduodenal tube, 100 ml

Ingredients:

Tobramycin sulphate	1.22 g

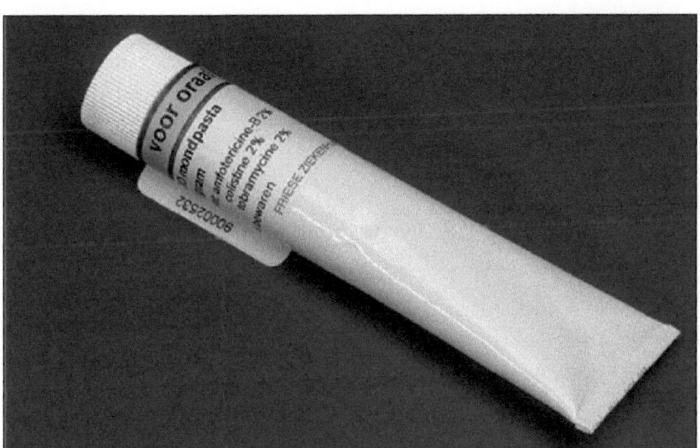

Fig. 5.4 The oral paste for SDD

Colistin sulphate	1 g
Amphotericin B	5 g
Methyloxybenzoate 15% in propylene glycol	0.5 ml
Polysorbate 80	0.8 ml
Purified water	to give 100 ml

Packaging material:
PET bottle 100 ml with a polyethylene Dosepac screw cap (see Fig. 5.5).

Each 10 ml of the suspension contains:

Amphotericin B	500 mg
Colistin sulphate	100 mg
Tobramycin (as -sulphate)	80 mg

Storage temperature: between 4 °C and 8 °C
Stability: 6 months

c. SDD suppository
Ingredients:

Amphotericin B	200 mg
Colistin sulphate	100 mg
Tobramycin sulphate	61 mg
Adeps solidus (Witepsol H15)	1,845 mg

Packaging material:
Plastic single unit suppository container of 2.3 ml (see Fig. 5.6).

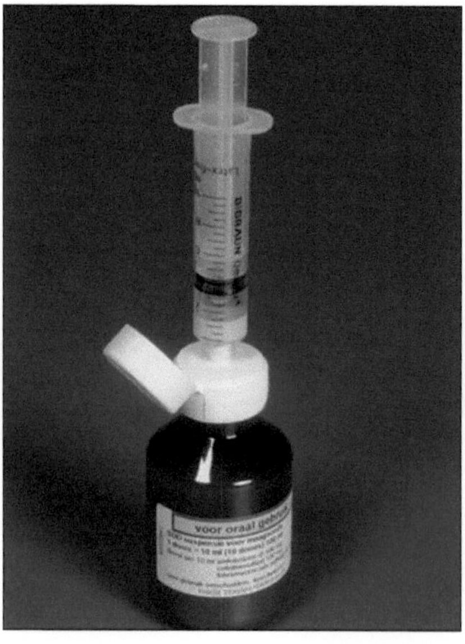

Fig. 5.5 The SDD suspension for use in gastroduodenal tube

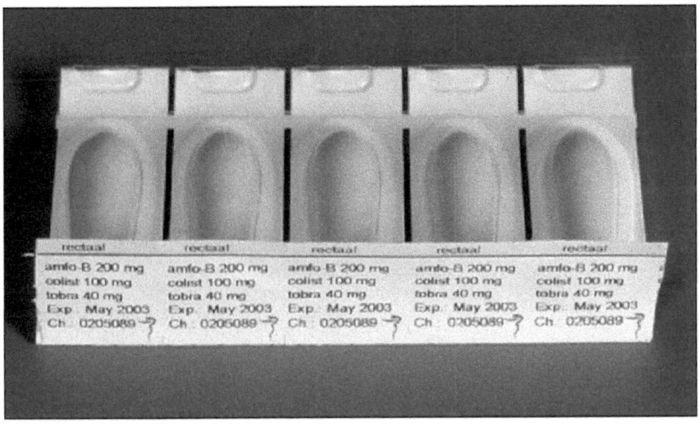

Fig. 5.6 The SDD suppository

The suppository contains:

Amphotericin B	200 mg
Colistin sulphate	100 mg
Tobramycin (sulphate)	40 mg

Storage temperature: between 4ºC and 8ºC
Stability: 12 months

Precautions:
In the process of compounding a formulation such as those mentioned above, manufacturing personnel should wear protective gowns, protective gloves and protective respiratory equipment.
The handling of the active substances should preferably be done in a biohazard safety cabinet.
The choice of the personal protective equipment is based upon the hazard evaluation of the work environment, i.e. the active substances. Information about the health risks of working with the active ingredients may be found in the corresponding Material Safety Data Sheets (MSDS) [28].

Quality Control of Drugs for SDD

When controlling the quality of manufactured drugs for SDD, the laboratory testing should be conducted in the context of GMP, and more specifically in accordance with good control laboratory practice (GCLP). There are several analytical techniques that can be used for quality control of the drugs for SDD. The same analyses can be applied when testing the stability of the preparations. Stability testing is necessary to determine the shelf-life and storage conditions of the drugs. In the literature, data concerning quality control and stability testing of drugs containing amphotericin B, colistin sulphate and tobramycin sulphate is sparse. Amphotericin B can be determined by HPLC analysis or

UV–spectroscopy; colistin concentrations can be assessed by HPLC; and tobramycin can be determined by enzyme immunoassay [29–35].

References

1. De Jonge E, Schultz MJ, Spanjaard L et al (2003) Effects of selective decontamination of digestive tract on mortality and acquisition of resistant bacteria in intensive care: a randomised controlled trial. Lancet 362:1011-1016
2. Lode H, Höffken G, Kemmerich B et al (1992) Systemic and endotracheal antibiotic prophylaxis of nosocomial pneumonia in ICU. Intensive Care Med 18 [Suppl 1]:24-27
3. Kimura A, Mochizuki T, Nishizawa K et al (1998) Trimethoprim-sulfamethoxazole for the prevention of methicillin-resistant Staphylococcus aureus pneumonia in severely burned patients. J Trauma 45:383-387
4. Sirvent JM, Torres A, El-Ebiary M et al (1997) Protective effect of intravenously administered cefuroxime against nosocomial pneumonia in patients with structural coma. Am J Respir Crit Care Med 155:1729-1734
5. Nathens AB, Marshall JC (1999) Selective decontamination of the digestive tract in surgical patients: a systematic review of the evidence. Arch Surg 134:170-176
6. D'Amico R, Pifferi S, Leonetti C et al (1998) Effectiveness of antibiotic prophylaxis in critically ill adult patients: systematic review of randomised controlled trials. BMJ 316:1275-1285
7. Hurley JC (1995) Prophylaxis with enteral antibiotics in ventilated patients: selective decontamination or selective cross-infection? (PMID: 7786000) Antimicrob Agents Chemother 39:941-947
8. Kollef MH (1994) The role of selective digestive tract decontamination on mortality and respiratory tract infections. A meta-analysis. Chest 105:1101-1108
9. Heyland DK, Cook DJ, Jaeschke R et al (1994) Selective decontamination of the digestive tract. An overview. Chest 105:1221-1229
10. Selective Decontamination of the Digestive Tract Trialists' Collaborative Group (1993) Meta-analysis of randomised controlled trials of selective decontamination of the digestive tract. BMJ 307:525-532
11. Vandenbroucke-Grauls CM, Vandenbroucke JP (1992) Effect of selective decontamination of the digestive tract on respiratory tract infections and mortality in the intensive care unit. Lancet 338:859-862
12. van Saene HK, Stoutenbeek CP, Hart CA (1991) Selective decontamination of the digestive tract (SDD) in intensive care patients: a critical evaluation of the clinical, bacteriological and epidemiological benefits. J Hosp Infect 18:261-277
13. Korinek AM, Laisne MJ, Nicolas MH et al (1993) Selective decontamination of the digestive tract in neurosurgical intensive care unit patients: a double-blind, randomized, placebo-controlled study. Crit Care Med 21:1466-1473
14. Silvestri L, Milanese M, Oblach L et al (2002) Enteral vancomycin to control methicillin-resistant Staphylococcus aureus outbreak in mechanically ventilated patients. Am J Infect Control 30:391-399
15. de la Cal MA, Cerdá E, van Saene HK et al (2004) Effectiveness and safety of enteral vancomycin to control endemicity of methicillin-resistant Staphylococcus aureus in a medical/surgical intensive care unit. J Hosp Infect 56:175-183
16. Cerdá E, Abella A, de la Cal MA et al (2007) Enteral vancomycin controls methicillin-resistant Staphylococcus aureus endemicity in an intensive care burn unit: a 9-year prospective study. Ann Surg 245:397-407
17. Taxis K, Barber ND (1993) Ethnographic study of incidence and severity of intravenous drug errors. BMJ 326 (7391):684

18. Department of Health (2001) Building a safer NHS for patients. London: Stationery Office
19. Institute of Medicine Committee on the Quality of Health Care in America (2000) To err is human. Washington: National Academy Press
20. Thur MP, Miller WA, Latiolais CJ (1972) Medication errors in a nurse-controlled parenteral admixture program. Am J Hosp Pharm 29:298-304
21. Hartley GM, Dhillon S (1998) An observational study of the prescribing and administration of intravenous drugs in a general hospital. Int J Pharm Pract 6:38-45
22. O'Hare, MCB, Gallagher T, Shields MD (1995) Errors in the administration of intravenous drugs. BMJ 310:1536-1537
23. Clark CM, Bailie GR, Whitaker AM et al (1986) Parenteral drug delivery—value for money? Pharm J 236:453-455
24. Brennan TA, Leape LL, Laird N et al (1991) Incidence of adverse events and negligence in hospitalized patients. N Engl J Med 324:370-376
25. Leape LL, Brennan TA, Laird N et al (1991) The nature of adverse events in hospitalized patients. N Engl J Med 324:377-384
26. Gawande A (2002) Complications. New York: Metropolitan Books, Henry Holt & Co
27. Taylor FO (March 1947) Quality control. J Am Pharm Assoc III (3)
28. MSDS database at http://www.ohsah.bc.ca
29. Le Brun PPH, Graaf AI de, Vinks AATMM (2000) A high performance liquid chromatographic method for the determination of colistin in serum. Ther Drug Monit 22:589-593
30. Trissel LA (2000) Stability of Compounded Formulations 2nd edn. Washington DC: American Pharmaceutical Association
31. Wilkinson JM, McDonald C, Parkin JE et al (1998) A high-performance liquid-chromatography assay for amphotericin B in a hydrophilic colloidal paste base. J Pharm Biomed Anal 17:751-755
32. Dentinger PJ, Swenson CF, Anaizi NH (2001) Stability of amphotericin B in an extemporaneously compounded oral suspension. Am J Health-Syst Pharm 58:1021-1024
33. Lue LP, Hadman ST, Vancura A (2002) Liquid chromatographic determination of amphotericin B in different pharmaceuticals. J AOAC Int 85:15-19
34. Feron B, Adair CG, Gorman SP et al (1993) Interaction of sucralfate with antibiotics used for selective decontamination of the gastrointestinal tract. Am J Hosp Pharm 50:2550-2553
35. Li J, Milne RW, Nation RL et al (2003) Stability of colistin and colistin methanesulfonate in aqueous media and plasma as determined by high-performance liquid chromatography. Antimicrob Agents Chemother 47:1364-1370

Suggested readings

Medicinal products for human and veterinary use: Good manufacturing practices. Commission Directive 2003/94/EC. Strasbourg: Council of Europe, 2003

Quality in the manufacture of medicines and other healthcare products (2000) Sharp J. London: Pharmaceutical Press

Guidance for Industry Q7A Good Manufacturing Practice Guidance for active pharmaceutical ingredients. Rockville MD: ICH, 2001

European Pharmacopoeia Fifth Edition. Strasbourg: Council of Europe, 2005

The United States Pharmacopoeia 29th Edition. Rockville, MD: United States Pharmacopeial Convention, 2006

GMP Hospital Pharmacy. The Hague: Dutch Association of Hospital Pharmacists (NVZA), 1998

PIC/S Guide to good practices for preparation of medicinal products in pharmacies. Draft 2. Geneva: PIC/S, 2006.

Chapter 6
Nursing and Practical Aspects in the Application and Implementation of SDD

Jetske Oenema and Jeanine Mysliwiec

Introduction

In our book, as far as the practice of SDD is concerned, the role of the nurse is of paramount importance. Unless all nurses are individually trained in the proper application of the oral paste decontamination will be unsuccessful. Conversely, persistent or repeated unsuccessful decontamination should lead to a study of precisely how the SDD paste is applied by the nursing staff, which can lead to additional training. The introduction and implementation of SDD at the bedside is mainly the task of a senior nurse, and in daily practice the intensive care nurses play an important part, as they are the ones who actually administer the medication. The goals of SDD are shown in Table 6.1.

The following description of the introduction of SDD in the ICU in the Leeuwarden Medical Centre, a 24-bed mixed medical and surgical ICU within a regional Dutch hospital, illustrates the role of the nurse in the complete process.

SDD in Practice

Selective eradication of potential pathogenic microorganisms (PPM) in the oral cavity and decontamination of the rest of the digestive tract are achieved by the application of nonabsorbable antibiotics (e.g. polymyxin E, tobramycin and amphotericin B) into the mouth/throat and the gut. A nasogastric tube is used to apply 10 ml suspension containing 100 mg polymyxin E, 80 mg tobramycin and 500 mg amphotericin B (4 times a day). In addition, early respiratory infections during the ICU stay, which can be caused by commensal respiratory flora on admission, are prevented by the use of systemic antibiotics. During the early days in the ICU, eradication of PPM in the mouth/throat and the rest of the digestive tract is not yet established. In our ICU we use 1 g cefotaxime i.v. 4 times daily for the first 4 days. In the case of proven allergy to cephalosporins, i.v. ciprofloxacin 400 mg twice daily is given for 4 days instead of cefotaxime.

In the case of (suspected) MRSA, vancomycin 500 mg is added to the SDD

Table 6.1 Goals of selective decontamination of the digestive tract (SDD)

Goal	Measure
Selective eradication of PPMs in the oral cavity	Sticky paste (such as Orabase®) containing nonabsorbable antibiotics (e.g. polymyxin E, tobramycin and amphotericin B) applied in the mouth/throat, four times a day
Decontamination of the rest of the digestive tract	SDD solution applied via the gastric tube, four times a day. If a duodenal tube is used, 50% of the SDD volume is given via the gastric tube and 50% via the duodenal route Sticky paste around tracheostomy, if present, four times a day
Decontamination of special sites	SDD suppositories in blind loops, two to four times a day Antibiotics by nebuliser to eliminate colonisation of the trachea Regular changing of gastric tubes, urinary catheters, tracheal cannulas, central lines, and other indwelling catheters
Prophylaxis to prevent respiratory infections that may occur early during ICU stay, caused by commensal respiratory flora	Systemic antibiotics (cefotaxime) for 4 days
Prevention of cross-contamination	Hand hygiene
Monitoring the effectiveness of SDD	Regular cultures (surveillance) of throat swabs and faeces (rectal swabs)

suspension and vancomycin 2% to the orabase. Although the surveillance cultures can switch from positive to negative for MRSA, this cannot be seen as a reliable indication that MRSA has genuinely been eradicated from the gut.

Implementation

Before implementing SDD in the unit, it is important to know what materials are required, to find out where they can be ordered and how they will be supplied. Both the pharmacist and the ICU nurses on the wards need a broad orientation concerning the materials. A combined exploration of the possibilities is preferable. The focus should be on availability, effectiveness and cost.

What materials are needed?

- Chlorhexidine solution
- SDD paste
- SDD suspension
- Mouth swabs
- NaCl 0.9% 20cc
- (Possibly) SDD suppositories

Administration of SDD Paste and Suspension

Upper Gastrointestinal Tract

The way the SDD suspension is manufactured in the hospital pharmacy may show some variation. It may be delivered to the ward as powder that should be made into a suspension, it may be a suspension of polymyxin and tobramycin, in which case the intensive care nurses should add the amphotericin B, or it may be delivered as a complete 'ready-to-use' solution. However, once the suspension is complete the administration is the same.

First, clean the mouth thoroughly. Suction any excess saliva and remove remains of SDD paste applied earlier with a mouth swab and chlorhexidine. The teeth should also be cleaned (if applicable).

Secondly, apply a small amount of paste (varying in volume between that of a pea and that of a bean) inside the mouth using a mouth swab or finger. It is important that the paste is evenly applied throughout the mouth, including the buccal cavity, the upper and lower jaw and the cheeks and tongue. If the patient is awake, SDD can be applied to the tongue; patients can do this themselves.

The patient should then receive 10 cc of a 2% SDD suspension administered via the nasogastric tube, which is subsequently flushed with 20 cc NaCl 0.9%. Nasogastric tubes on free drainage should be clamped for 1 hour. The suspension can be given in combination with other oral medication providing the tube is flushed between administrations.

If the patient has a nasogastric and a jejunostomy tube, 5 cc suspension is given via the nasogastric tube and 5 cc via the jejunostomy catheter, allowing both the stomach and the postpyloric parts of the bowel to be decontaminated. Patients without a nasogastric tube can drink the suspension, but the amphotericin B means it is anything but appetising.

Lower Gastrointestinal tract

The lower gastrointestinal tract should be decontaminated by means of the PTA suspension, which is given by gastric or duodenal tube. To ensure it reaches the rectum, early and effective defaecation is necessary. All intestinal exits (anus, ileostomy, colostomy) that are continuous with the stomach are reached in this way.

Administration of SDD Suppositories

Patients with an ileostomy or colostomy are given the suppository rectally and via the stoma. The suppositories should adequately decontaminate all closed bowel loops. Enemas can also be used. Both suppositories and enemas should contain 2% PTA. Any bowel loops that will be reached by the gastric suspension do not need suppositories providing the bowel motility is intact and the patient passes faeces.

If indicated, the suppository can be given vaginally, in particular to decrease *Candida* colonisation (to prevent urinary tract infection). The key issue is that SDD is administered everywhere that colonisation with potentially pathogenic microorganisms may occur. Parenteral administration of cefotaxime will not be discussed here.

Tracheostomy

In patients with a tracheostomy, we apply the oral SDD-paste (containing 2% polymyxin E, 2% tobramycin and 2% amphotericin B) around the stoma (2–4 times a day) in addition to the other SDD and hygienic measures. Tracheostomy patients are at particularly high risk of exogenous infections, and despite rigorous hygiene measures in the control group, topical application of SDD paste was shown to reduce exogenous respiratory infections in tracheotomised patients in an ICU [1]. First, residual SDD paste is removed from the tracheal stoma. Secondly, the tracheal stoma is cleaned with a chlorhexidine solution. Thirdly, the new paste is applied around the tracheal stoma. In addition, the tracheal cannula is changed for a new one every week, as a thin layer of microorganisms can adhere to the tracheal cannula leading to on-going colonisation and respiratory infection.

Aerosol

In case of PPMs in the tracheal aspirate, medication should be administered by aerosol to eliminate this abnormal colonisation. For AGNB, polymyxin E 2% 5 ml or tobramycin 40—80 mg (i.v. solution) in 5 ml can be used four times daily. For Gram-positive microorganisms (for instance *S. aureus*) a first-generation cephalosporin (e.g. cephradine) 500 mg can be given by aerosol four times daily. Yeasts and *Aspergillus* can be eliminated by amphotericin B 5 mg four times daily in 5 ml. Usually this therapy is continued until two consecutive cultures of tracheal aspirate no longer show the target microorganism.

Supplying Medication and Materials

Medication

The medication is supplied by the hospital pharmacy and should become part of the ward's stock. Previously on our unit it was supplied individually for each patient, but this created problems, as the paste can only be stored for a short period of time and must be kept refrigerated and used immediately after removal from the refrigerator. Multiple patients can benefit from the same bottle of SDD suspension. The frequency of deliveries depends on the expiry date and the amount required (how many patients are being treated and the dosage prescribed for each). To arrange for the right amount of SDD to be on the ward it is advisable to find out the mean number of patients who are being treated by SDD at the same time. Multiplying that number by 40 ml gives the mean volume of SDD suspension that is needed per day in the unit.

Additional Materials and Storage

The hospital's stores supply mouth swabs. Trial and error finally revealed which was the best option.

Storage is an important issue because of the limited shelf-life of most of the preparations needed. It was decided that a separate shelf in the refrigerator should be used for the SDD medication, where it could be arranged in plain view.

Which Are the Patients for Whom SDD is Indicated?

The exact indication may vary due to local protocols. The aim is to decontaminate patients who are at risk of acquiring PPMs leading to secondary endogenous infections. The time-frame chosen depends on the local protocol. Usually patients who are expected to be mechanically ventilated for more than 36 hours and patients who are expected to be treated in the ICU for more than 72 hours (with or without mechanical ventilation) are decontaminated.

Surveillance samples
Samples taken from body sites where bacteria are usually carried (throat/gut), with the aim of detecting carrier status.

Diagnostic samples
Samples from body sites that are normally sterile (lower airways, bladder, blood), with the aim of diagnosing infection and to evaluating efficacy of parenteral/enteral antibiotics.

Culture Sample Collection

On admission

In order to recognise and record any existing infections and colonisation, culture samples are taken immediately on admission to the unit. Both surveillance and diagnostic samples are taken at this time. SDD can then be started. Samples are taken of all body materials that can be obtained at this time. Samples are taken from the throat and rectum to determine any pathologic colonisation and/or carriage. Sputum, urine, and wound and drain fluids are taken to detect infection, as these sites are usually sterile. In the postoperative patient, it may not be necessary to obtain drain fluid samples when such cultures have been obtained in the operating room.

During Admission

Table 6.2 shows the surveillance samples that are collected twice weekly. The surveillance samples include specimens from ileostomies and colostomies. Usually the samples are taken on Mondays and Thursdays. However, if a patient is admitted on Sunday or Wednesday, it is not necessary to repeat sampling the next day. The samples can be obtained in the early morning (6:00 a.m.) to allow them to reach the microbiology laboratory early, or later in the morning when the patients are washed. Sputum and tracheostomy fluid are also cultured twice weekly. Strictly speaking, these are diagnostic samples and not surveillance samples, but because of the crucial information they can yield in the critical care setting they are taken routinely rather than on an "as indicated" basis.

Table 6.2 Surveillance samples to be collected twice weekly

Body material	Samples taken	Material used	Remarks
Throat	Twice weekly	Swab	Surveillance
Rectum	Twice weekly	Swab	Surveillance
Ileo-/colostomy	Twice weekly	Swab	Surveillance
Sputum	Twice weekly	Sputum culture pot	Surveillance/diagnostic
Tracheostomy	Twice weekly	Swab	Surveillance/diagnostic
Urine	On admission	Urine sample	Diagnostic and as indicated
Wound	Twice weekly	Swab	Surveillance/diagnostic
Drain fluid	Twice-weekly	Swab or sample	Diagnostic
Blood	As indicated	Sample	Diagnostic
Other	As indicated	Swab or sample	Diagnostic

Diagnostic samples of urine and blood are only taken on admission and as indicated. Urine remains uncontaminated with the use of SDD. "Other diagnostic samples" include drain site openings, for example. Samples are taken from both rectum and ileostomies/colostomies.

Microbiology Request forms

Because more than one sample is taken from each patient, several forms normally have to be used. We have therefore developed a standard form on which multiple requests can be entered, to reduce the workload and simplify the system.

Cooperation With the Microbiology Laboratory

The delivery of a large number of samples to a microbiology laboratory elsewhere in the hospital or even outside the hospital requires good cooperation between the two departments concerned.

We have found it possible to agree on the following points:

- Use of a single request form
- Delivery of samples to the laboratory early in the day, e.g. before 10:00 a.m.

This enables users to minimise the workload and avoid delays in obtaining test results.

Swabs for Sample Collection: Wet vs Dry

Samples are collected using cotton swabs. These can be used in two ways, either moistened with NaCl 0.9% or dry. In our daily practice virtually all culture sites are wet to some degree, and we obtain adequate culture results without moistening the cotton swabs.

Persistent Microorganisms in Throat and Rectal Swabs

When surveillance cultures persistently show Gram-negative colonisation in the throat, resistance and application should be checked. When bacteria are sensitive to tobramycin and/or polymyxin E the method of applying the SDD paste should be re-assessed. In addition, the gastric tube should be removed and a new one inserted. The oral paste can be applied eight times daily until the throat is properly decontaminated.

To achieve decontamination in the rectal cultures, gastric emptying and defaecation should be aggressively promoted by prokinetic medication (e.g.

erythromycin) and laxatives (polyethylene glycol or neostigmin). It is hardly ever necessary to increase the amount of SDD suspension given by gastric tube.

An Example of a Local Set-Up in a Regional Hospital ICU

In the year 2000, when we first started using SDD, our ICU capacity was 11 beds. We had 35.1 full time-equivalent intensive care nurses. The patients were mixed medical and surgical patients with a mean APACHE II score of 19.5. Around 600 admissions a year for a mean stay of 6 days were counted. In the first year 220 patients received SDD, for a total of 2,812 treatment days.

The Working Group

A working group was set up before SDD was introduced in the unit. The following disciplines were represented:
Intensivist
Unit manager
ICU nurse
Microbiologist

Study Day

SDD was incorporated into our annual study day programme. The ICU nurse representing the work group explained the practical implementation of SDD, and each ICU nurse was issued with a protocol.

Instruction

Instruction in the procedure was given in the form of "on-the-job training". A small group of nurses received intensive schooling, and these subsequently passed on their knowledge to their colleagues.

Workload

The intensive care nurses were initially reluctant to see SDD introduced, the main reasons for this being the increased workload and the lack of time for extra procedures. However, after approximately six months the positive effect of SDD began to show and resistance to it subsided. Positive aspects for the intensive care nurses were the decrease in purulent sputum and the obvious decrease in secondary pneumonia. This resulted in a decline in the frequency of suctioning of the trachea, from routinely four times daily to twice daily. In addition, patients no longer suffered from halitosis! The absence of any resistant strain requiring isolation nursing and of outbreaks since the start of SDD has actually significantly reduced the workload for all members of staff in the ICU.

Timing of Administration of SDD

SDD should be applied four times a day. The administration times coincide with those for regular nursing interventions; this is advantageous for both the patient and the nurse, as the patient is not unduly disturbed and the nurse can incorporate SDD into the regular nursing care and/or regular administration of medication.

SDD can therefore be given at 0900 hours, 1500 hours, 2100 hours and 0300 hours. Night-time doses are slightly flexible, so as to correspond with periods when the patient is awake. It must be realised that some medications, e.g. sucralfate, inactivate the SDD suspension; the concurrent administration of such medications should be avoided.

Hygiene Measures

Hygiene is an essential part of SDD, and a high level of basic hygiene should therefore exist in the unit. Some of the most basic rules that should be applied are:

1. General hygiene: the wearing of jewellery and watches should be forbidden.
2. Hand hygiene: sterilisation alcohol hand-wash should be used after washing hands with water and soap. This procedure should be available at each bedside. Gloves should be easily available and are used for any contact with body fluids. Whenever there is any physical contact with the patient, whether by a nurse or another colleague, an apron should be worn.
3. All patients can be washed with hibiscrub to prevent skin colonisation from being the harbinger of another colonisation. However, this will mainly apply to colonisation with Gram-positive bacteria such as *S. aureus*.
4. Every effort should be made to avoid any one nurse being in contact with many different patients during the same shift. This might be achieved by allocating one nurse to one or a maximum of two different patients.
5. It is obligatory to remove all indwelling catheters (gastric tubes and urinary catheters) regularly, e.g. once a week, to prevent colonisation and subsequent infection.

Patients' Experiences

Much has been said about the introduction of SDD to the unit and the consequences of this, but how does the patient experience it? Sedated patients and short-stay patients seem to be relatively unaffected by administration of the SDD paste. They grimace a little, indicating that the taste is unpleasant. Long-stay patients, however, whether sedated or conscious, find it particularly unpleasant, become nauseous and occasionally vomit. It is difficult to convince these patients of the benefits of SDD.

Conclusion

The implementation of SDD needs a multidisciplinary approach. All staff should be aware of the background and the importance of all aspects. Therefore, the nursing staff should be closely involved in the implementation and introduction of SDD to the intensive care unit.

Acknowledgements. We thank M.J. Schultz and P.E. Spronk for providing Table 6.1 and some lines of text.

References

1. Morar P, Makura Z, Jones A et al (2000) Topical antibiotics on tracheostoma prevents exogenous colonization and infection of lower airways in children. Chest 117:513-518

Chapter 7
The Effects of Hand-Washing, Restrictive Antibiotic Use and SDD on Morbidity

Markus J. Schultz and Peter E. Spronk

Introduction

Considerable numbers of critically ill patients suffer from infections during their stay in the intensive care unit (ICU), as outlined in Chapter 3. The most common infections in these patients are lower respiratory tract infections (e.g., ventilator-associated pneumonia; VAP), followed by infections of the urinary tract and bloodstream infections [1]. The treatment of infections in critically ill patients is difficult. First, a steady increase in the prevalence of antibiotic resistance among microorganisms has made the treatment of infections more complex [2] and no breakthroughs for new antibiotic classes are in sight at present. Secondly, although it is speculated that the high incidence of infections in critically ill patients may be the result of the underlying disease and/or immunoparalysis (as may develop in the course of sepsis), therapy aimed at modulation of the immune response during infection is further from clinical practice than before [3, 4]. The prevention of infection and control may be a more effective strategy in intensive care medicine than the treatment of infections.

Hand-washing and restrictive use of antibiotics have long been the two major interventions in infection control in intensive care medicine [5, 6]. Hand-washing would be an effective measure to prevent transmission of pathogens via the hands of healthcare workers. According to this theory, the source of pathogens is thought to be the ICU environment, including other colonised or infected critically ill patients. Restrictive use of antibiotics would control the emergence of antibiotic resistance by reducing the antibiotic load. In this approach, antibiotics are to be used only when infection is established on admission or firmly diagnosed during stay on ICU. The efficacy of both interventions has been questioned [7, 8].

As long as 20 years ago, Stoutenbeek et al. advocated another approach to the prevention of infections in the ICU than antibiotic treatment and/or immunotherapy [9]. This so-called *selective decontamination of the digestive tract* (SDD) is a more proactive approach, which tries to eradicate potential pathogens from the gut, leaving patients' own indigenous microflora intact to maintain optimal colonisation resistance. SDD is aimed primarily at the prevention of VAP in critically ill patients. However, other infections are also prevented.

In this chapter, we will first discuss the ineffectivity of hand-washing and restrictive use of antibiotics in infection control in the ICU. After this, we will focus on the effects of SDD in intensive care medicine on morbidity. We will discuss briefly why and how SDD can be an effective measure to prevent nosocomial infections in critically ill patients, and how SDD is applied. Finally, we will discuss the literature on the efficacy of SDD in preventing VAP and bacteraemia in mixed intensive care patients and in specific patient populations. Although SDD is also used for the prevention of gut-derived infections in liver transplantation patients, this is beyond the scope of the present chapter, and the reader is referred to Chapter 13.

Efficacy of Hand-Washing and Restrictive Use of Antibiotics in Critically Ill Patients

The two interventions that have been the cornerstone of infection control in intensive care medicine up to now have never been adequately tested for their efficacy; neither have they been proven not to be effective in the ICU setting. Indeed, the effect of hand-washing on infection rate has never been evaluated in randomised trials, although it is still highly recommended by experts as one of the cornerstones of infection prevention. Restrictive antibiotic use may have effects on the prevention of resistant microorganisms. However, restrictive antibiotic regimens have been tested in critically ill patients and failed to show a beneficial effect in infection prevention. The prompt initiation of adequate antibiotic treatment for critically ill patients has been shown to reduce mortality and is thus at odds with restrictive use [10].

Efficacy of Hand Hygiene

As long ago as in 1861, it was demonstrated that hand hygiene can directly improve survival [11]. Indeed, Semmelweis confirmed that implementation of hand-washing with chlorinated lime reduced mortality from 'childbed fever' from 11% to 3% (historical controls were used). Since *S. pyogenes* is a high-level pathogen, it is not surprising that hand-washing reduced mortality. However, it should be borne in mind that Semmelweis, in his time, was studying the effects of hand hygiene in an extreme situation: histopathologists working with necrotic tissue in the mortuary also delivered babies. In addition, general hygiene standards in his time were different from those we have today, so that one might develop some scepticism about hand hygiene [8]. Unfortunately, neither properly designed trials evaluating the effect of hand hygiene on pneumonia and septicaemia in critically ill patients [12] nor studies evaluating whether fewer critically ill patients die when healthcare workers adhere to stringent hand hygiene have been performed [13]. Nonetheless, hand hygiene is still the only measure that is highly recommended [5, 14].

Critically ill patients develop overgrowth in their throat and gut of $>10^9$ PPM/ml of saliva or gram of faeces. Intense contact with those patients may lead to contamination of the hands to levels of $>10^6$ PPM per square centimetre of finger surface area [15]. For hand hygiene to be effective disinfecting agents are required and the hand-washing procedure must take at least 2 min. Only then are contamination levels lowered, and at most by 10^4 PPM per square centimetre of finger surface, which still leaves up to 10^2 per square centimetre of finger surface. However, compliance with hand hygiene procedures is low. With high-level pathogens, such as *Salmonella*, *Shigella*, rotavirus and *E. coli* 0157, there is generally low-level carriage, with $<10^3$ enteric pathogens per gram of faeces [16, 17]. Thus, in such cases hand hygiene can be effective. Indeed, studies have shown that hand hygiene controls outbreaks with these pathogens [16, 17], and Semmelweis' publication on *S. pyogenes* is another good example of this [11]. Unfortunately, this strategy will not work in the situation in which there is a large reservoir of pathogens, as there is of PPM in critically ill patients. Furthermore, under the hypothetical circumstances of completely clearing hand contamination, hand hygiene could never exert an influence on the other major infection problem in critically ill patients, i.e. primary endogenous infections: hand hygiene also fails to clear oropharyngeal and gastrointestinal carriage and/or overgrowth of potentially pathogenic microorganisms present on arrival in the ICU.

Keeping these considerations in mind, high standards of hygiene, including hand hygiene, are part of the SDD infection control protocol. This will lead to a reduction in the level of hand contamination, transmission of pathogens, and exogenous infections.

Restrictive Use of Antibiotics

As well as hand-washing, restrictive antibiotic usage in ICU patients has been thought to be effective in infection control in ICU medicine. 'Restrictive antibiotic usage' in this context means that antibiotics should only be used when the presence of infection is confirmed by microbiological methods. With a focus on VAP, several invasive techniques for establishing the diagnosis of VAP have been introduced in the past [18]. Interestingly, from recent studies it can be concluded that invasive strategies and subsequent restrictive antibiotic usage may not work at all [19, 20]. Moreover, delaying adequate parenteral antibiotic treatment on ICU admission while trying to establish a microbiological diagnosis has been shown to increase mortality in ICU patients with VAP and sepsis [21]. SDD has shown to be a strategy with less systemic antibiotic use than routine antibiotic strategies [10, 22]. However, the topical, including oral, administration of antibiotics means that a larger total amount of antibiotics is used than would otherwise be the case; this might theoretically lead to higher costs and to more resistant microorganisms. These two issues are discussed in Chapters 9 and 10.

Pathogens That Are a Threat to Critically Ill Patients

Critically ill patients are at risk of life-threatening infections. Only a limited range of (potentially) pathogenic microorganisms (PPM) contributes to morbidity in these patients. SDD aims to eradicate patient's carrier status for these pathogens, leaving patient's own indigenous flora intact. In Chapter 2 these PPMs are discussed with their corresponding intrinsic pathogenicity indices.

What Kind of Infections Do They Cause?

To understand the effect of SDD on morbidity, it is mandatory to be familiar with the concept. We will briefly summarise the concept here, while in Chapter 2 this item is discussed more in detail. In the SDD terminology, three types of infection are recognised: *primary endogenous* infections, *secondary endogenous* infections, and *exogenous* infections. Microorganisms that are not present in the patient's flora on admission but are within the environment of the ICU are first acquired in the oropharynx. In the critically ill patient, oropharyngeal acquisition leads to secondary carriage in the gut. Consequently, this may lead to colonisation of and subsequent overgrowth in normally sterile internal organs, such as the lower airways, where these pathogens cause infections (so-called *secondary endogenous* infections). In contrast to the *secondary endogenous* infections, in *exogenous* infections, pathogens are also acquired on the unit, but have never been present in the throat and/or gut flora of the patient, i.e. infection was not preceded by colonisation. This type of infection is due to breaches of hygiene and can occur at any time during a patient's stay in the ICU. Finally, *primary endogenous* infections are due to microorganisms that are carried into the ICU by the patient; that is to say that these pathogens were present in their flora on admission as part of their carrier status. The goal of SDD is to prevent, or eradicate if initially present, oropharyngeal and gastrointestinal carriage of PPMs, especially hospital PPMs, while leaving the indigenous flora, which is thought to provide some protection against overgrowth with resistant bacteria, largely undisturbed [9].

Effectiveness of SDD in Preventing Infections in Critically Ill Patients

In this overview we discuss the nine prospective randomised studies in which the complete original SDD protocol (PTA by oral and intestinal routes in combination with cefotaxime i.v.) is compared with controls (no oral or intestinal antibiotics and no parenteral antibiotic) for the end-point lower airway infection (Table 7.1) [23–31]. The ten meta-analyses, which include all prospective studies that have been published, will then be discussed. Most of the RCTs have focused on the prevention of VAP; some of them also determined the effect of SDD on bacteraemia in the critically ill. What follows here is a short presentation of the individual studies.

In the first prospective randomised study on SDD, Kerver et al. determined whether prevention of colonisation with Gram-negative microorganisms reduced the incidence of Gram-negative bacterial infections [23]. Ninety-six critically ill patients were randomised to receive either the original oral and intestinal SDD with cefotaxime, or standard therapy (control). In the SDD group, no colonisation with Gram-negative bacteria was found, whereas there was an elevated incidence of Gram-negative colonisation in the oropharynx, the respiratory tract and the digestive tract in the control group. In addition, significantly more nosocomial infections were diagnosed in the control group than in the SDD group; in particular, there was a higher incidence of respiratory tract infections and bacteraemia. Mortality from an acquired infection was significantly less frequent in the SDD group.

Table 7.1 Outcomes of prospective randomised trials–respiratory tract infections

Author/s [ref.]	No. in SDD group–control group	% Incidence of pulmonary infection (SDD vs control)	*p*-Value
Kerver et al. [24]	49–47	12 vs 85	<0.01
Blair et al. [27]	161–170	10 vs 34	0.002
Tetteroo [25]	56–58	1 vs 8	<0.05
Rocha et al. [29]	47–54	15 vs 46	<0.001
Palomar et al. [32]	50–49	17 vs 50	0.005
Jacobs et al. [30]	45–46	0 vs 9	<0.05
Verwaest et al. [33][a]	200–185	25 vs 34	<0.05
De la Cal [30]	58–59	18 vs 26	0.03
Stoutenbeek [31]	201–200	62 vs 100	<0.01

[a]Two study groups were compared with one control group; see text

In the same year as the study just mentioned, another one on the efficacy of SDD in reducing respiratory tract infections was published [24]. In this stratified, randomised, prospective study, 331 patients were recruited over an 18-month period, with 256 patients remaining >48 hours in the ICU. Stratification by acute physiology and chronic health evaluation (APACHE II) preceded randomisation to standard treatment (standard antibiotic therapy) or SDD (polymyxin, amphotericin, tobramycin and i.v. cefotaxime). The incidence of nosocomial infection was significantly lower in the SDD group than in the control group. Those patients with admission APACHE II scores of 10–19 demonstrated the most significant reduction in nosocomial infection.

In 1990, Tetteroo studied 112 patients undergoing oesophageal resection over a two-year period [25]. The medication was started before surgery and continued for ten days after surgery. The treatment group also received metronidazol on the day of surgery. This huge study showed a significant decrease in colonisation and infection as a result of SDD.

In 1994, two studies were published on the use of the original SDD in critically ill patients [26, 27]. Rocha et al. [26] studied 101 patients who randomly received SDD or placebo. These patients all spent more than three days on mechanical ventilation during stays of more than five days in the unit and were free of infection at the start of the study. There was a significantly lower incidence of bacteraemia and respiratory tract infections in the SDD group than in placebo-treated patients. Jacobs et al., in the same year, confirmed the positive effects of this SDD regimen on the incidence of respiratory tract infections in critically ill patients, although in their study it was not possible to demonstrate a reduction in the incidence of bacteraemia [27]. This may be explained by the remarkably low baseline infection rate relative to those in other SDD studies.

In 1997, two studies on SDD were published [28, 29]. Verwaest compared patients treated with the original SDD components with placebo-treated patients and with a group receiving ofloxacin [28]. The limited decrease in infection rate in the SDD-treated patients is completely at odds with observations recorded in all the other trials. For instance, Palomar found a highly significant reduction in lower airway infections in the same year [29].

With the exception of the Verwaest publication, it has consistently been shown that the classic SDD regimen with PTA, administered both in the oral paste form and as the gastrointestinal suspension, plus i.v. cefotaxime, provides strong protection against respiratory tract infections and bloodstream infections. Remarkably, the incidence of VAP in the control groups varied from 9% [27] to 85% [23]. One possible reason for this wide variation is variation in patient populations. Another is the application of different methods of diagnosing pneumonia. In some studies the diagnosis of VAP was made on clinical, radiological and microbiological criteria alone. It can be argued that in these studies the reduction in respiratory tract infections is in fact a reduction in colonisation and purulent tracheobronchitis and not a reduction in pneumonia. Other studies used bronchoscopic techniques, with quantitative cultures, which usually indicate an incidence of VAP that is half that found when the diagnosis is made on clinical, radiological and microbiological criteria. Nonetheless, even in these studies, the SDD regimen was still followed by a significantly lower incidence of pneumonia than was conventional treatment. In addition, it has been recently shown that tracheal aspirate and bronchoalveolar lavage are both equally useful as diagnostic tools in the critically ill patient to diagnose pneumonia [18]. The reduction of VAP in studies with both the classic and other antimicrobial combinations is shown in the meta-analyses that will be discussed below.

Efficacy of SDD Seen in Meta-Analyses

Over 20 years of clinical research on SDD have generated fifty-six RCTs, which have been assessed in ten meta-analyses [32–41], half of them from Europe (all from Italy) and half from North America (two are from Canada and three from the United States). All but one meta-analysis [38] assessed the efficacy of SDD in mixed ICU-populations (Table 7.2).

Table 7.2 Ten meta-analyses of randomised controlled trials [RCTs] of selective digestive decontamination [SDD]: morbidity data (RCTs, randomised controlled trials; SDD, selective decontamination of the digestive tract; NR, not reported; AGNB, aerobic Gram-negative bacilli; G+, Gram-positive bacteria; #, risk difference; ‡, relative risk)

Author(s) [ref.]	Year	Number of RCTs	Aggregate number	Endpoints	Odds ratio	95% confidence interval
SDD Trialists Collaborative Group [38]	1993	22	4,142	Pneumonia	0.33	0.27–0.40
Kollef [39]	1994	16	2,270	Pneumonia	0.145#	0.116–0.174
Heyland et al. [40]	1994	25	3,395	Pneumonia	0.46‡	0.39–0.56
D'Amico et al. [41]	1998	33	5,727	Pneumonia	0.35	0.29–0.41
Nathens et al. [42]	1999	11	NR (surgical)	Pneumonia	0.19	0.15–0.26
				Bacteraemia	0.51	0.34–0.75
			NR (medical)	Pneumonia	0.45	0.33–0.62
				Bacteraemia	0.77	0.43–1.36
Redman et al. [43]	2001	NR	NR	Pneumonia	0.31	0.20–0.46
Safdar et al. [44]	2004	4	259 (liver transplant)	Infection overall	0.88‡	0.73–1.09
				Infection due to AGNB	0.16‡	0.07–0.37

Continue →

Continue **Table 7.2**

Author(s) [ref.]	Year	Number of RCTs	Aggregate number	Endpoints	Odds ratio	95% confidence interval
Liberati et al. [45]	2004	36	6,922	Pneumonia	0.35	0.29–0.41
Silvestri et al. [46]	2005	42	6,075	Fungal carriage	0.32	0.19–0.53
				Fungal infections	0.30	0.17–0.53
				Fungaemia	0.89	0.16–4.95
Silvestri et al. [47]	2007	51	9,230	Bloodstream infections	0.63	0.46–0.87
				Bloodstream infections due to AGNB	0.44	0.19–0.73
				Bloodstream infections due to G+	0.92	0.59–1.44

Of the ten meta-analyses, seven had pneumonia as the primary end-point. The end-points in the other three meta-analyses were yeast carriage and infection, bloodstream infections (BSI) and infections in liver transplant patients. Table 7.2 summarises the results of all ten meta-analyses. All meta-analyses of SDD that reported pneumonia as an outcome measure found a beneficial effect. The most recent Cochrane meta-analysis, published in 2004 and involving 6,922 patients, showed that SDD using parenteral and enteral antimicrobials reduces the odds ratio for pneumonia to 0.35 (95% CI 0.29–0.41) [39]. On average, five patients need to receive SDD to prevent one case of pneumonia. A total of 9,230 patients were available for the first meta-analysis of RCTs in which BSI were reported [41]. SDD using parenteral and enteral antimicrobials significantly reduced the odds ratio for BSI to 0.63 (95% CI 0.46–0.87). Additionally, a protective effect against BSI due to AGNB was found, with an odds ratio of 0.44 (95% CI 0.27–0.73) [41].

The Effect of SDD on Morbidity in Specific Patient Populations

In addition to the studies in critically ill patients, SDD has been applied in other specific patient populations. Burn patients and liver transplant patients are discussed in Chapters 13 and 14. At this point we will discuss miscellaneous indications, including cardiac failure and cardiac surgery, upper gastrointestinal tract surgery, neurosurgery and pancreatitis.

1. Cardiac and cardiac surgical patients. In these patients, it is postulated that a reduction in the endotoxin load of the digestive tract will reduce the systemic inflammatory response. SDD reduces endotoxin load, which has several favourable effects in patients with heart failure or cardiac surgery [42–44]. Some studies do not show a beneficial effect [45]. This discrepancy concerning endotoxin load can be explained: the negative studies did not use the optimal mix of antimicrobial agents. The strongest reduction (10^4) in faecal endotoxins is reached when the combination of polymyxin and tobramycin is used. The current literature on endotoxin binding has recently been well summarised elsewhere [46] and is also dealt with in Chapter 12.

Concerning clinical outcomes, Fox found in a before-and-after study of cardiac surgery patients that the incidence of infection was not reduced by SDD but that mortality, as the primary outcome parameter, was significantly lower in the SDD group [47]. In addition, Flaherty found a reduced incidence of infection in cardiac surgery patients, with less need of systemic antibiotics but no significant effect on mortality [48]. In conclusion, in the cardiac and cardiac surgery patient population, the endotoxin load can be reduced by the use of tobramycin and polymyxin and a limited number of studies have shown benefit in terms of clinical outcome.

2. Patients with upper gastrointestinal tract surgery. Patients undergoing oesophageal and gastric surgery have been studied in two trials. Schardey found in a RCT involving 200 patients that infections (in particular pneumonia) were significantly less frequent [49]. Oesophagointestinal dysfunction occurred only in patients who had not undergone decontamination. The need for antibiotic therapy was significantly lower in the SDD group, and reinterventions showed a trend towards reduced incidence in this group. In 114 patients after oesophageal resection, Tetteroo also found that pulmonary infections and wound infections were significantly reduced [25]. Another study involving 25 patients treated with SDD and 70 who did not receive SDD showed less frequent infections, shorter periods of mechanical ventilation and shorter stays in intensive care in the SDD group, though none of these differences achieved statistical significance. The potency of this study may have been too low for significant differences on these outcome measurements to be detected [50].

3. Neurology and neurosurgery patients. This specific population was studied in three trials. Korinek showed that 96 patients treated with SDD had significantly less pneumonia, urinary tract infections and sinusitis than the 95 patients not treated with SDD [51]. However, the parenteral part of the SDD (3rd-generation cephalosporin) was not part of the study protocol. Jacobs, in 1992, could not find any significant effect of SDD on infection prevention owing to a very low incidence of infection in the control group [27].

Gosney showed in 203 patients who had suffered acute stroke that those who underwent SDD developed significantly lower rates of pneumonia than the placebo group (7 versus 1; $p = 0.029$) [52].

4. Pancreatitis patients. The only study on SDD in patients with pancreatitis was published in 1995 [53] and compared 50 patients treated with SDD against 52 placebo treated patients. The SDD treated patients had a lower incidence of infection and a lower mortality rate and also underwent fewer laparotomies.

Conclusions, and Outstanding Questions

Taken together, the results of the individual studies indicate a strong protective effect of SDD against VAP and bacteraemia, from which ICU patients can die. But is mortality influenced by use of SDD? The reduction of mortality in ICU patients is the topic of Chapter 8 of this book. Secondly, is SDD cost effective? Although only a minority of studies looked at costs, and the reduction of costs by the application of SDD in particular, some conclusions can be drawn from the present literature (see Chapter 10). Finally, the risk of antimicrobial resistance must be discussed: is this a real problem with the use of SDD, or does SDD prevent the development and spread of antibiotic resistance? This issue is dealt with in Chapter 11. The reader is referred to these chapters for further reading on these topics.

References

1. Vincent JL, Bihari DJ, Suter PM et al (1995) The prevalence of nosocomial infection in intensive care units in Europe. Results of the European Prevalence of Infection in Intensive Care (EPIC) Study. EPIC International Advisory Committee. JAMA 274:639-644
2. Kollef MH, Sherman G, Ward S et al (1999) Inadequate antimicrobial treatment of infections: a risk factor for hospital mortality among critically ill patients. Chest 115:462-474
3. van der Poll T (2001) Immunotherapy of sepsis. Lancet Infect Dis 1:165-174
4. Schultz MJ, van der Poll T (2002) Modulation of pulmonary innate immunity during bacterial infection: animal studies. Arch Immunol Ther Exp 50:159-167
5. Larson EL (1995) APIC guideline for handwashing and hand antisepsis in health care settings. Am J Infect Control 23:251-269
6. Paterson DL (2003) Restrictive antibiotic policies are appropriate in intensive care units. Crit Care Med 31:S25-28
7. Van Saene HK, Petros AJ, Ramsay G et al (2003) All great truths are iconoclastic: selective decontamination of the digestive tract moves from heresy to level 1 truth. Intensive Care Med 29:677-690
8. Silvestri L, Petros AJ, Sarginson RE et al (2005) Handwashing in the intensive care unit : a big measure with modest effects. J Hosp Infect 2005:59:172-179
9. Stoutenbeek CP, van Saene HK, Miranda DR et al (1984) The effect of selective decontamination of the digestive tract on colonisation and infection rate in multiple trauma patients. Intensive Care Med 10:185-192
10. de Jonge E, Schultz MJ, Spanjaard L et al (2003) Effects of selective decontamination of digestive tract on mortality and acquisition of resistant bacteria in intensive care: a randomised controlled trial. Lancet 362:1011-1016
11. Semmelweis IP (1861) Die Aetiologie, der Begriff und die Prophylaxis des Kindbettfiebers. Pest: Hartleben

12. Daschner FD, Frey P, Wolff G et al (1982) Nosocomial infections in intensive care wards: a multicenter prospective study. Intensive Care Med 8:5-9
13. Larson E (1999) Skin hygiene and infection prevention: more of the same or different approaches? Clin Infect Dis 29:1287-1294
14. Jarvis WR (1994) Handwashing—the Semmelweis lesson forgotten? Lancet 344:1311-1312
15. Salzman TC, Clark JJ, Klemm L (1967) Hand contamination of personnel as a mechanism of cross-infection in nosocomial infections with antibiotic-resistant Escherichia coli and Klebsiella-Aerobacter. Antimicrobial Agents Chemother 7:97-100
16. Khan MU (1982) Interruption of shigellosis by hand washing. Trans R Soc Trop Med Hyg 76:164-168
17. Tarr PI (1995) Escherichia coli O157:H7: clinical, diagnostic, and epidemiological aspects of human infection. Clin Infect Dis 20:1-8; quiz 9-10
18. Heyland D, Dodek P, Muscedere J et al (2006) A randomized trial of diagnostic techniques for ventilator-associated pneumonia. N Engl J Med 355:2619-2630
19. Fagon JY, Chastre J, Wolff M et al (2000) Invasive and noninvasive strategies for management of suspected ventilator-associated pneumonia. A randomized trial. Ann Intern Med 132:621-630
20. Ruiz M, Torres A, Ewig S et al. (2000) Noninvasive versus invasive microbial investigation in ventilator-associated pneumonia: evaluation of outcome. Am J Respir Crit Care Med 162:119-125
21. Alvarez-Lerma F (1996) Modification of empiric antibiotic treatment in patients with pneumonia acquired in the intensive care unit. ICU-Acquired Pneumonia Study Group. Intensive Care Med 22:387-394
22. van der Voort PHJ, van Roon EN, Kampinga GA et al (2004) A before–after study of multiresistance and cost of selective decontamination of the digestive tract. Infection 32:271-277
23. Kerver AJ, Rommes JH, Mevissen-Verhage EA et al (1988) Prevention of colonization and infection in critically ill patients: a prospective randomized study. Crit Care Med 16:1087-1093
24. Blair P, Rowlands BJ, Lowry K et al (1991) Selective decontamination of the digestive tract: a stratified, randomized, prospective study in a mixed intensive care unit. Surgery 110:303-309; discussion 309-310
25. Tetteroo GWM, Wagenvoort JHT, Castelein A et al (1990) Selective decontamination to reduce gram-negative colonisation and infections after oesophageal resection. Lancet 335:704-707
26. Rocha LA, Martin MJ, Pita S et al (1992) Prevention of nosocomial infection in critically ill patients by selective decontamination of the digestive tract. A randomized, double blind, placebo-controlled study. Intensive Care Med 18:398-404
27. Jacobs S, Foweraker JE, Roberts SE (1992) Effectiveness of selective decontamination of the digestive tract in an ICU with a policy encouraging a low gastric pH. Clin Intensive Care 3:52-58
28. Verwaest C, Verhaegen J, Ferdinande P et al. (1997) Randomized, controlled trial of selective digestive decontamination in 600 mechanically ventilated patients in a multidisciplinary intensive care unit. Crit Care Med 25:63-71
29. Palomar M, Alvarez-Lerma F, Jorda R, Bermejo B (1997) Prevention of nosocomial infection in mechanically ventilated patients: selective digestive decontamination versus sucralfate. Clin Intensive Care 8:228-235
30. de la Cal MA, Cerda E, Garcia-Hierro P, van Saene HK et al (2005) Survival benefit in critically ill burned patients receiving selective decontamination of the digestive tract: a randomized, placebo-controlled, double-blind trial. Ann Surg 241:424-430
31. Stoutenbeek CP, van Saene HKF, Little RA et al (2007) The effect of selective decontamination of the digestive tract on mortality in multiple trauma patients: a multicenter randomized controlled trial. Intensive Care Med 33:261-270
32. Selective Decontamination of the Digestive Tract Trialists' Collaborative Group (1993) Meta-analysis of randomised controlled trials of selective decontamination of the digestive

tract. BMJ 307:525-532
33. Kollef MH (1994) The role of selective digestive tract decontamination on mortality and respiratory tract infections: a meta-analysis. Chest 105:1101-1108
34. Heyland DK, Cook DJ, Jaeschke R et al (1994) Selective decontamination of the digestive tract: an overview. Chest 105: 1221-1229
35. D'Amico R, Pifferi S, Leonetti C et al (1998) Effectiveness of antibiotic prophylaxis in critically ill adult patients: systematic review of randomised controlled trials. BMJ 316:1275-1285
36. Nathens AB, Marshall JC (1999) Selective decontamination of the digestive tract in surgical patients: a systematic review of the evidence. Arch Surg 134:170-176
37. Redman R, Ludington E, Crocker M et al (2001) Analysis of respiratory and non-respiratory infections in published trials of selective decontamination (abstract). Intensive Care Med 27 [Suppl 1]: S128
38. Safdar N, Said A, Lucey MR (2004) The role of selective digestive decontamination for reducing infection in patients undergoing liver transplantation: a systematic review and meta-analysis. Liver Transpl 10:817-827
39. Liberati A, D'Amico R, Pifferi S et al (2004) Antibiotic prophylaxis to reduce respiratory tract infections and mortality in adults receiving intensive care. Cochrane Database Syst Rev [1]:CD000022
40. Silvestri L, van Saene HKF, Milanese M et al (2005) D. Impact of selective decontamination of the digestive tract on fungal carriage and infection: systematic review of randomised controlled trials. Intensive Care Med 31:898-910
41. Silvestri L, van Saene HKF, Milanese M et al (2007) Selective decontamination of the digestive tract reduces bacterial bloodstream infection and mortality in critically ill patients. Systematic review of randomised, controlled trials. J Hosp Infect 65:187-203
42. Conraads VM, Jorens PG, De Clerck LS et al (2004) Selective intestinal decontamination in advanced chronic heart failure: a pilot trial. Eur J Heart Fail 6:483-491
43. Martinez-Pellus AE, Merino P, Bru M et al (1993) Can selective digestive decontamination avoid the endotoxemia and cytokine activation promoted by cardiopulmonary bypass? Crit Care Med 21:1684-1691
44. Marinez-Pellus AE, Merino P, Bru M et al (1997) Endogenous endotoxemia of intestinal origin during cardiopulmonary bypass. Role of type of flow and protective effect of selective digestive decontamination. Intensive Care Med 23:1251-1257
45. Bouter H, Schippers EF, Luelma SA et al (2002) No effect of preoperative selective gut decontamination on endotoxemia and cytokine activation during cardiopulmonary bypass: a randomized, placebo-controlled study. Crit Care Med 30:38-43
46. Oudemans-van Straaten HM, van Saene HK, Zandstra DF (2003) Selective decontamination of the digestive tract: use of the correct antibiotics is crucial. Crit Care Med 31:334-335
47. Fox MA, Peterson S, Fabri BM et al (1991) Selective decontamination of the digestive tract in cardiac surgery patients. Crit Care Med 19:1486-1490
48. Flaherty J, Nathan C, Kabins SA et al (1990) Pilot trial of selective decontamination for prevention of bacterial infection in an intensive care unit. J Infect Dis 162:1393-1397
49. Schardey HM, Joosten U, Finke U et al (1997) The prevention of anastomotic leakage after total gastrectomy with local decontamination. Ann Surg 225:172-180
50. Riedl S, Peter B, Geiss HK et al (2001) Microbiological and clinical effects of selective bowel decontamination in transthoracic resection of carcinoma of the esophagus and cardia. Chirurg 72:1160-1170
51. Korinek AM, Laisne MJ, Nicolas MH et al (1993) Selective decontamination of the digestive tract in neurosurgical intensive care patients: a double blind, randomized, placebo-controlled study. Crit Care Med 21:1466-1473
52. Gosney M, Martin MV, Wright AE (2006) The role of selective decontamination of the digestive tract in acute stroke. Age Ageing 35:42-47
53. Luiten EJ, Hop WC, Lange JF et al (1995) Controlled clinical trial of selective decontamination for the treatment of severe acute pancreatitis. Ann Surg 222:57-65

Chapter 8
The Effects of SDD on Mortality

Evert de Jonge

Introduction

Chris Stoutenbeek introduced selective decontamination of the digestive tract (SDD) in intensive care medicine in 1984 [1]. Since than, fifty-six RCTs have been performed, with different end-points. Two of them did not report mortality data. This chapter will focus on the main twenty-eight prospective, randomised studies on *mortality* in intensive care patients that have been published [2–29]. In addition, the meta-analyses on mortality will be discussed. In thirtheen of the published studies the effects of decontamination of both the oral cavity and the rest of the gastrointestinal tract in combination with systemic prophylaxis were investigated [2–13, 29], while eight studies investigated the effects of decontamination of the oral cavity and gastrointestinal tract [14–21], four studies investigated oral decontamination only [23-26], one study examined combined oral decontamination with systemic prophylaxis [22] and four studies investigated the effects of intestinal decontamination only [27, 28, 30, 31]. The published studies not only differed in the combinations of topical and systemic prophylaxis, but also showed wide variations in the antimicrobial agents used. The original SDD schedule (polymyxin, tobramycin, amphotericin combined with cefotaxime) was used in eight studies. In other studies cefotaxime was replaced by ceftriaxone, trimethoprim, ofloxacin, ciprofloxacin or ceftazidime. Tobramycin was sometimes replaced by gentamicin, neomycin, nalidixic acid or norfloxacin. Nystatin sometimes replaced amphotericin B, and in some studies no antifungal agent was given at all. Moreover, in some studies vancomycin was added to the topical agents [32]. In this chapter, we will summarise the effects of the different SDD regimens on mortality among ICU patients.

Studies Using Both Topical and Systemic Prophylaxis

In fourteen studies the influence of the combination of topical and systemic antibiotics on mortality of ICU patients was investigated. In one of these studies oropharynged antibiotics were the only topical treatment [22], in the other 13 studies both oropharynged and intestinal decontamination were applied. The effects of SDD on survival are summarized in Table 8.1. One of the studies showed a significant reduction in overall mortality in ICU patients who were artificially ventilated for more than three days, had an ICU stay of at least five days and had no infection on enrolment in the study [9]. If an analysis is made on an intention-to-treat basis, the difference in mortality is of borderline significance (RR 0.70, 95% CI 0.49-1.02) In the study conducted by Krueger [7], mortality was lower in a subgroup of 237 surgical patients who had APACHE II scores in the midrange stratum (APACHE II scores of 20–29 on ICU admission). In these patients ICU mortality was 33% in the placebo group, as against 16.4% in the SDD group ($p = 0.01$). Analysis of their entire study population yielded a nonsignificant reduction in mortality (relative risk 0.76; $p = 0.13$ by Cox proportional hazards modelling). Interestingly, had the data been analysed on a strict intention-to-treat basis, the reduction in mortality would have been significant (relative risk of 0.69, 95% CI 0.51–0.95). Recently, we presented the findings of the largest single-centre randomised controlled trial on the use of the classic SDD regimen (polymyxin E, tobramycin, amphotericin B and cefotaxime) in 934 surgical and medical ICU patients [29]. We found lower ICU mortality (odds ratio 0.60, 95% CI 0.42–0.82) and lower hospital mortality (odds ratio

Table 8.1 Summary of SDD studies using the combination of topical and systemic antibiotics. Relative risks (RR) and number needed to treat (NNT) to prevent one death are calculated using the data as originally published

First author [ref.]	No. of patients	RR for mortality	NNT
Abele-Horn [22]	88	1.12 (0.42–2.96)	–
Aerdts [2]	88	0.71 (0.25–2.01)	17
Blair [3]	256	0.79 (0.49–1.28)	26
Cockerill [4]	150	0.57 (0.25–1.28)	15
Jacobs [5]	79	0.62 (0.37–1.05)	5
De Jonge [29]	934	0.69 (0.49–0.85)	12
Kerver [6]	96	0.90 (0.49–1.65)	30
Krueger [7]	527	0.76 (0.53–1.09)	11
Palomar [8]	99	0.98 (0.52–1.83)	175
Rocha [9]	101	0.48 (0.26–0.89)	4
Sanchez-Garcia [10]	271	0.84 (0.63–1.11)	12
Ulrich [11]	112	0.69 (0.47–1.03)	6
Verwaest [12]	660	1.11 (0.79–1.56)	–36
Winter [13]	183	0.83 (0.58–1.19)	14

0.71, 95% CI 0.53–0.94) in patients treated with the original SDD protocol using PTA enterally and cefotaxime parenterally. The lower mortality was found in both surgical and medical patients. The more pronounced reduction in mortality found in this trial relative to the pooled results of previous studies included in the meta-analyses may be related to the fact that SDD patients were not mixed with control patients in the same ICUs. Instead of this, SDD patients and control patients were treated in separate units, preventing the transfer of potential pathogenic bacteria from control patients to SDD patients and the exogenous infections this could otherwise have caused.

Over recent years several meta-analyses of the SDD studies have been performed. The first meta-analysis that suggested that SDD might reduce mortality was published in 1993 by the SDD Trialists' Collaborative Group [33]. In their pooled analysis of all studies they found an odds ratio for mortality of 0.80 (95% CI 0.67–0.97) for patients treated with a combination of topical and systemic antibiotics. Subsequent meta-analyses have confirmed these findings. The Italian Cochrane group reported an odds ratio of 0.80 (95% CI 0.69–0.93) for mortality in patients treated with topical and systemic antibiotics [34], and a meta-analysis by Nathens et al. [35] reported lower mortality for surgical patients (odds ratio 0.60, 95% CI 0.41–0.88) and a trend towards lower mortality in medical patients (odds ratio 0.75, 95% CI 0.53–1.06). We can conclude that many studies were too low in power to detect a reduction in mortality by SDD, but that the pooled data nonetheless show that mortality is indeed lower in patients treated with a combination of topical and systemic agents. However, the use of meta-analyses has been the subject of substantial criticism. Some of them were based on studies that had never been published and had thus never passed the peer-review process [32]. Furthermore, the methodological quality of the individual studies has been questioned. The result of a meta-analysis depends, among other things, on the quality of the studies included. Van Nieuwenhoven's finding that the effect of SDD on the incidence of pneumonia was inversely related to the methodological quality of the study was alarming. Reassuringly, no such relation was found between mortality and trial quality [36]. Nevertheless, meta-analyses are not universally accepted as evidence and the use of SDD to lower mortality in ICU patients has remained highly controversial. In summary, there is evidence from a meta-analysis that mortality is lower in SDD-treated patients [34, 35]; there is a study reporting significantly improved survival following SDD [29]; and, finally, there is one study that has revealed improved survival in the subgroup of patients in the midrange stratum of APACHE II scores and overall improved survival if the data are analysed on a strict intention-to-treat basis [7]. We can conclude that there is sufficient evidence to justify the opinion that the classic SDD regimen combining systemic prophylaxis with oropharyngeal and intestinal decontamination can reduce mortality in ICU patients. The only study that compared systemic plus oropharyngeal antibiotics only (without intestinal decontamination) against control [22] did not find a reduction in mortality.

SDD Using Only Topical Antibiotics

A number of trials studied the effect of topical prophylaxis on mortality in ICU patients. These studies compared oropharyngeal decontamination, intestinal decontamination, or oropharyngeal and intestinal decontamination combined against no prophylaxis (Table 8.2). None of these studies showed improved survival in SDD-treated patients. When an analysis is made of the pooled data, there appears to be no benefit of SDD in the studies applying intestinal or combined oropharyngeal and intestinal antibiotics. Although not statistically significant, a trend towards increased survival is seen in the studies using oropharyngeal

Table 8.2 Summary of SDD trials comparing the effects of topical antibiotics only on mortality (*combination of topical and systemic antibiotics was compared with systemic treatment, RR relative risk for mortality, CI confidence interval)

First author [ref.]	No. of patients	Antibiotics	Relative risk (95% CI)
Oropharyngeal decontamination vs control			
Bergmans [23]	226	PGVan	0.75 (0.51–1.12)
Laggner [24]	67	GA	0.66 (0.33–1.32)
Pugin [25]	52	PneoVan	0.98 (0.47–2.04)
Rodriguez-Roldan [26]	28	PTA	0.87 (0.35–2.14)
Pooled data	*403*		*0.77 (0.58–1.04)*
Intestinal decontamination vs control			
Brun-Buisson [27]	133	PneoNal	0.98 (0.51–1.86)
Cerra [28]	48	NysNor	1.20 (0.66–2.18)
Gaussorgues [30]	118	PGAVan	1.00 (0.69–1.44)
Godard [31]	181	PTA	0.69 (0.34–1.40)
Pooled data	*480*		*0.95 (0.72–1.26)*
Intestinal and oropharyngeal decontamination vs control			
Ferrer [14]	101	PTA*	1.05 (0.57–1.94)
Hammond [15]	239	PTA*	1.05 (0.59–1.87)
Lingnau [16]	357	PTA, PCiproA, Cipro*	1.27 (0.70–2.3)
Gastinne [17]	445	PTA	1.10 (0.87–1.39)
Korinek [18]	191	PTAVan	1.28 (0.73––2.25)
Quinio [19]	148	PGA	1.15 (0.53–2.50)
Unertl [20]	39	PGA	0.88 (0.32–2.40)
Wiener [21]	61	PGNys	0.76 (0.42–1.37)
Pooled data	*1581*		*1.09 (0.91–1.30)*

decontamination only. The absence of a beneficial effect in the trials using topical prophylaxis only may be due to the fact that early infections are not prevented by SDD that does not include initial systemic antibiotics [37]. On the basis of these results, it is stressed that SDD should be administered according to the complete and original protocol, with PTA enterally and cefotaxime parenterally.

Severity of Illness and the Effects of SDD

Whereas SDD including both topical and systemic antibiotics appears to improve mortality in ICU patients, it is not clear whether all ICU patients or only specific subgroups of patients will benefit from SDD. Several studies have looked at the influence of severity of illness on the effects of SDD. Sun and others reported that the relative risk reduction for mortality was highest in the SDD studies with the highest mortality in the control group, suggesting that SDD was most beneficial in patients with highest severity of illness [38]. Krueger et al. reported lower mortality in the midrange stratum with APACHE II scores of 20–29 (relative risk 0.51, 95% CI 0.30–0.88). In the stratum with low APACHE II scores they found a (nonsignificant) relative risk for mortality of 0.885 (95% CI 0.47–1.66) and in the very small subgroup with APACHE II scores higher than 30 ($n = 49$), a relative risk of 1.59 (95% CI 0.77–3.3) [7]. In contrast, in the 1998 Cochrane meta-analysis, the extent of the treatment effect was quite consistent across all severity groups [34]. In our study in 934 patients [29], we too found lower mortality in all risk groups (unpublished analysis).

Effects of SDD in Surgical and Medical Patients

In their meta-analysis of SDD studies published in 1999, Nathens et al. analysed medical and surgical patients separately [35]. They reported a statistically significant decrease in mortality in all surgical patients treated with SDD, whereas no difference was found in medical patients. However, as outlined above, the beneficial effects of SDD appear to be present only if the full SDD protocol is applied, i.e. with the combination of topical and systemic antibiotics. In Nathens' analysis of studies using the combination of systemic and topical treatment the odds ratio for mortality was 0.60 (95% CI 0.41–0.88) in surgical patients and 0.75 (95% CI 0.53–1.06), suggesting that the treatment effects may not be different in surgical and medical patients. Similar results were found in the Cochrane analysis, with a somewhat lower odds ratio for mortality in surgical patients compared with medical patients but with considerable overlap of the 95% confidence intervals [34].

Effects of SDD in Specific Subgroups of Patients

SDD has also been studied in prospective, randomised trials in specific subgroups other than ICU patients. Tetteroo et al. studied SDD vs standard perioperative antibiotic prophylaxis in patients undergoing elective oesophageal resection for carcinoma [39]. In this randomised study, SDD resulted in a reduction in pneumonia and wound infections. Mortality was very low and was not altered by SDD (2% vs 3%). Another randomised trial addressed the influence of SDD on outcome after total gastrectomy. SDD was started the day before surgery and included both topical and systemic prophylaxis; it resulted in reduced frequencies of anastomotic leaks and pneumonia. Mortality tended to be lower in the SDD-treated patients (4.9%, as against 10.6%; $p = 0.1$) [40].

In a prospective, randomised trial of SDD in acute pancreatitis, Luiten et al. demonstrated a reduction in the incidence of pneumonia and infected pancreatic necrosis, associated with a decrease in mortality (22%, as against 35%) [41]. In this study SDD was compared with no antibiotic prophylaxis. No data are available for comparison of SDD with systemic antibiotic prophylaxis, which is presently considered to be standard treatment for necrotic pancreatitis [42].

Four relatively small randomised trials conducted in patients undergoing liver transplantation have been published. Although most of these trials showed a reduction in the incidence of infections, none of them showed improved survival [43–47] However, owing to the small number of patients included in these trials and the low mortality in the control groups, these studies clearly had inadequate potency to exclude a survival benefit in SDD-treated patients. SDD for patients undergoing liver transplantation is discussed more in detail in Chapter 13.

SDD has also been studied in patients who have just undergone heart surgery. None of the published studies showed improved survival in the treated patients [48–50]. As mortality is very low in this subgroup of patients (4–7% in one of these trials), thousands of patients per treatment group would be necessary for a survival benefit in SDD-treated patients to be obvious.

Effects of SDD on Mortality Compared with Other Interventions

According to the meta-analysis performed by d'Amico et al. [34], the combination of topical and systemic antibiotics would reduce mortality in ICU patients from 28.2% to 24.1%, representing an absolute risk reduction of 4.1%. In the largest single studies even higher absolute risk reductions were found (8.5% [7] and 8.1% [29]). This is very much comparable with the absolute risk reduction for mortality found for activated protein C in patients with severe sepsis (6.1%) [51] or corticosteroids in patients with septic shock (10%) [52]. However, whereas activated protein C and corticosteroids are indicated in only a very small population of ICU patients with either severe sepsis or septic shock not responding to ACTH, SDD could be given to all ICU patients who are expected to stay on the ventilator for at least two days or in the ICU for at least three days. During our SDD study, approximately 30% of all patients admitted to our ICU were included in the trial [29]. Accordingly, the potential impact on mortality for the entire ICU population is much higher for interventions that are applicable for large number of patients, such as SDD. In this respect, SDD is comparable to strict glucose control, which is associated with an absolute reduction in mortality of 3.4% but can be applied in the majority of ICU patients [53]. It highlights the immense importance that SDD may have for the care of critically ill patients [54].

Limitations of SDD

Although the precise mechanisms by which SDD may reduce mortality are largely unknown, it is generally agreed that SDD is active against aerobic Gram-negative bacteria but not against certain Gram-positive bacteria, such as methicillin-resistant *S. aureus* (MRSA) and vancomycin-resistant enterococci (VRE). The majority of SDD trials have been undertaken in hospitals with low incidences of MRSA and VRE. We cannot exclude the possibility that SDD would lead to an increased incidence of infections with MRSA and VRE in areas where these bacteria are endemic. Thus, the beneficial effects of SDD on mortality shown in different studies cannot be extrapolated to ICUs that have a high prevalence of these bacteria. It may be necessary to change the antibiotics included in the SDD regimen according to the endemic flora. Therefore, more studies are necessary before SDD can be advocated for units in which MRSA or VRE is endemic.

The use of antibiotics may lead to increased antimicrobial resistance. The emergence of resistance has not been shown in the published studies. However, the follow-up in those studies was not longer than 2-3 years and there is no guarantee that the widespread use of SDD will not lead to increased resistance over a longer period. Given the fact that no signs of increased resistance have been found so far, the fear of emerging resistance should not deter clinicians from giving a treatment that has been shown to reduce mortality in ICU patients. The issue of resistance is discussed in more detail in Chapter 9.

Conclusion

The results of individual studies and meta-analyses make it clear that patients benefit from SDD in terms of mortality when the complete and original protocol with PTA enterally and cefotaxime parenterally is used.

References

1. Stoutenbeek CP, van Saene HK, Miranda DR et al (1983) A new technique of infection prevention in the intensive care unit by selective decontamination of the digestive tract. Acta Anaesthesiol Belg 34:209-221
2. Aerdts SJ, van Dalen R, Clasener HA et al (1991) Antibiotic prophylaxis of respiratory tract infection in mechanically ventilated patients. A prospective, blinded, randomized trial of the effect of a novel regimen. Chest 100:783-791
3. Blair P, Rowlands BJ, Lowry K et al (1991) Selective decontamination of the digestive tract: a stratified, randomized, prospective study in a mixed intensive care unit. Surgery 110:303-309
4. Cockerill FR, Muller SR, Anhalt JP et al (1992) Prevention of infection in critically ill patients by selective decontamination of the digestive tract. Ann Intern Med 117:545-553
5. Jacobs S, Foweraker JE, Roberts SE (1992) Effectiveness of selective decontamination of the digestive tract in an ICU with a policy encouraging a low gastric pH. Clin Intensive Care 3:52-58
6. Kerver AJ, Rommes JH, Mevissen-Verhage EA et al (1988) Prevention of colonization and infection in critically ill patients: a prospective randomized study. Crit Care Med 16:1087-1093
7. Krueger WA, Lenhart FP, Neeser G et al (2002) Influence of combined intravenous and topical antibiotic prophylaxis on the incidence of infections, organ dysfunctions, and mortality in critically ill surgical patients: a prospective, stratified, randomized, double-blind, placebo-controlled clinical trial. Am J Respir Crit Care Med 166:1029-1037
8. Palomar M, Alvarez-Lerma F, Jorda R et al (1997) Prevention of nosocomial infection in mechanically ventilated patients: selective digestive decontamination versus sucralphate. Clin Intensive Care 8:228-235
9. Rocha LA, Martin MJ, Pita S et al (1992) Prevention of nosocomial infection in critically ill patients by selective decontamination of the digestive tract. A randomized, double blind, placebo-controlled study. Intensive Care Med 18:398-404
10. Sanchez Garcia M, Cambronero Galache JA, Lopez Diaz J et al (1998) Effectiveness and cost of selective decontamination of the digestive tract in critically ill intubated patients. A randomized, double-blind, placebo-controlled, multicenter trial. Am J Respir Crit Care Med 158:908-916
11. Ulrich C, Harinck-de Weerd JE, Bakker NC et al (1989) Selective decontamination of the digestive tract with norfloxacin in the prevention of ICU-acquired infections: a prospective randomized study. Intensive Care Med 15:424-431
12. Verwaest C, Verhaegen J, Ferdinande P et al (1997) Randomized, controlled trial of selective digestive decontamination in 600 mechanically ventilated patients in a multidisciplinary intensive care unit. Crit Care Med 25:63-71
13. Winter R, Humphreys H, Pick A et al (1992) A controlled trial of selective decontamination of the digestive tract in intensive care and its effect on nosocomial infection. J Antimicrob Chemother 30:73-87
14. Ferrer M, Torres A, Gonzalez J et al (1994) Utility of selective digestive decontamination in mechanically ventilated patients. Ann Intern Med 120:389-395
15. Hammond JM, Potgieter PD, Saunders GL et al (1992) A double-blind study of selective decontamination of the digestive tract in intensive care. Lancet 340:5-9
16. Lingnau W, Berger J, Javorsky F et al (1997) Selective intestinal decontamination in multiple trauma patients: prospective, controlled trial. J Trauma 42:687-694
17. Gastinne H, Wolff M, Delatour F et al (1992) A controlled trial in intensive care units of selective decontamination of the digestive tract with nonabsorbable antibiotics. The French Study Group on Selective Decontamination of the Digestive Tract. N Engl J Med 326:594-599
18. Korinek AM, Laisne MJ, Nicolas MH et al (1993) Selective decontamination of the digestive tract in neurosurgical intensive care unit patients: a double-blind, randomized, placebo-controlled study. Crit Care Med 21:1466-1473

19. Quinio B, Albanese J, Bues-Charbit M et al (1996) Selective decontamination of the digestive tract in multiple trauma patients. A prospective double-blind, randomized, placebo-controlled study. Chest 109:765-772
20. Unertl K, Ruckdeschel G, Selbmann HK et al (1987) Prevention of colonization and respiratory infections in long-term ventilated patients by local antimicrobial prophylaxis. Intensive Care Med 13:106-113
21. Wiener J, Itokazu G, Nathan C et al (1995) A randomized, double-blind, placebo-controlled trial of selective digestive decontamination in a medical-surgical intensive care unit. Clin Infect Dis 20:861-867
22. Abele-Horn M, Dauber A, Bauernfeind A et al (1997) Decrease in nosocomial pneumonia in ventilated patients by selective oropharyngeal decontamination (SOD). Intensive Care Med 23:187-195
23. Bergmans DC, Bonten MJ, Gaillard CA et al (2001) Prevention of ventilator-associated pneumonia by oral decontamination: a prospective, randomized, double-blind, placebo-controlled study. Am J Respir Crit Care Med 164:382-388
24. Laggner AN, Tryba M, Georgopoulos A et al (1994) Oropharyngeal decontamination with gentamicin for long-term ventilated patients on stress ulcer prophylaxis with sucralfate? Wien Klin Wochenschr 106:15-19
25. Pugin J, Auckenthaler R, Lew DP et al (1991) Oropharyngeal decontamination decreases incidence of ventilator-associated pneumonia. A randomized, placebo-controlled, double-blind clinical trial. JAMA 265:2704-2710
26. Rodriguez-Roldan JM, Altuna-Cuesta A, Lopez A et al (1990) Prevention of nosocomial lung infection in ventilated patients: use of an antimicrobial pharyngeal nonabsorbable paste. Crit Care Med 18:1239-1242
27. Brun-Buisson C, Legrand P, Rauss A et al (1989) Intestinal decontamination for control of nosocomial multiresistant gram-negative bacilli. Study of an outbreak in an intensive care unit. Ann Intern Med 110:873-881
28. Cerra FB, Maddaus MA, Dunn DL et al (1992) Selective gut decontamination reduces nosocomial infections and length of stay but not mortality or organ failure in surgical intensive care unit patients. Arch Surg 127:163-167
29. De Jonge E, Schultz MJ, Spanjaard L et al (2003) Effects of selective decontamination of the digestive tract on mortality and acquisition of resistant bacteria in intensive care: a randomised controlled trial. Lancet 362:1011-1016
30. Gaussorgues P, Salord F, Sirodot M et al (1991) Efficacies de la decontamination digestive sur la survenue des bactérémies nosocomiales chez les patients sous ventilation mécanique et recevant des bétamimétiques. Reanimation Soins Intensif Medecine d'Urgence 7:169-174
31. Godard J, Guillaume C, Reverdy ME et al (1990) Intestinal decontamination in a polyvalent ICU. A double-blind study. Intensive Care Med 16:307-311
32. Bonten MJ, Kullberg BJ, van Dalen R et al (2000) Selective digestive decontamination in patients in intensive care. The Dutch Working Group on Antibiotic Policy. J Antimicrob Chemother 46:351-362
33. Selective Decontamination of the Digestive Tract Trialists' Collaborative Group (1993) Meta-analysis of randomised controlled trials of selective decontamination of the digestive tract. BMJ 307:525-532
34. D'Amico R, Pifferi S, Leonetti C et al (1998) Effectiveness of antibiotic prophylaxis in critically ill adult patients: systematic review of randomised controlled trials. BMJ 316:1275-1285
35. Nathens AB, Marshall JC (1999) Selective decontamination of the digestive tract in surgical patients: a systematic review of the evidence. Arch Surg 134:170-176
36. van Nieuwenhoven CA, Buskens E, van Tiel FH et al (2001) Relationship between methodological trial quality and the effects of selective digestive decontamination on pneumonia and mortality in critically ill patients. JAMA 286:335-340
37. Baxby D, van Saene HK, Stoutenbeek CP et al (1996) Selective decontamination of the digestive tract: 13 years on, what it is and what it is not. Intensive Care Med 22:699-706

38. Sun X, Wagner DP, Knaus WA (1996) Does selective decontamination of the digestive tract reduce mortality for severely ill patients? Crit Care Med 24:753-755
39. Tetteroo GW, Wagenvoort JH, Castelein A et al (1990) Selective decontamination to reduce gram-negative colonisation and infections after oesophageal resection. Lancet 335:704-707
40. Schardey HM, Joosten U, Finke U et al (1997) The prevention of anastomotic leakage after total gastrectomy with local decontamination. A prospective, randomized, double-blind, placebo-controlled multicenter trial. Ann Surg 225:172-180
41. Luiten EJ, Hop WC, Lange JF et al (1995) Controlled clinical trial of selective decontamination for the treatment of severe acute pancreatitis. Ann Surg 222:57-65
42 Mitchell RM, Byrne MF, Baillie J (2003) Pancreatitis. Lancet 361:1447-1455
43. Smith SD, Jackson RJ, Hannakan CJ et al (1993) Selective decontamination in pediatric liver transplants. A randomized prospective study. Transplantation 55:1306-1309
44. Bion JF, Badger I, Crosby HA et al (1994) Selective decontamination of the digestive tract reduces gram-negative pulmonary colonization but not systemic endotoxemia in patients undergoing elective liver transplantation. Crit Care Med 22:40-49
45. Arnow PM, Carandang GC, Zabner R et al (1996) Randomized controlled trial of selective bowel decontamination for prevention of infections following liver transplantation. Clin Infect Dis 22:997-1003
46. Hellinger WC, Yao JD, Alvarez S et al (2002) A randomized, prospective, double-blinded evaluation of selective bowel decontamination in liver transplantation. Transplantation 73:1904-1909
47. Zwaveling JH, Maring JK, Klompmaker IJ et al (2002) Selective decontamination of the digestive tract to prevent postoperative infection: a randomized placebo-controlled trial in liver transplant patients. Crit Care Med 30:1204-1209
48. Bouter H, Schippers EF, Luelmo SA et al (2002) No effect of preoperative selective gut decontamination on endotoxemia and cytokine activation during cardiopulmonary bypass: a randomized, placebo-controlled study. Crit Care Med 30:38-43
49. Flaherty J, Nathan C, Kabins SA et al (1990) Pilot trial of selective decontamination for prevention of bacterial infection in an intensive care unit. J Infect Dis 162:1393-1397
50. Martinez-Pellus AE, Merino P, Bru M et al (1993) Can selective digestive decontamination avoid the endotoxemia and cytokine activation promoted by cardiopulmonary bypass? Crit Care Med 21:1684-1691
51. Bernard GR, Vincent JL, Laterre PF et al (2001) Efficacy and safety of recombinant human activated protein C for severe sepsis. N Engl J Med 344:699-709
52. Annane D, Sebille V, Charpentier C et al (2002) Effect of treatment with low doses of hydrocortisone and fludrocortisone on mortality in patients with septic shock. JAMA 288:862-871
53. Van den Berghe G, Wouters P, Weekers F et al (2001) Intensive insulin therapy in the critically ill patients. N Engl J Med 345:1359-1367
54. Aarts MA, Marshall JC (2002) In defense of evidence: the continuing saga of selective decontamination of the digestive tract. Am J Respir Crit Care Med 166:1014-1015

Chapter 9
Antimicrobial Resistance During 20 Years of Clinical SDD Research

Durk F. Zandstra, Hendrick K.F. van Saene and Peter H.J. van der Voort

Introduction

Selective decontamination of the digestive tract (SDD) is probably the most investigated clinical intervention in critically ill patients treated in intensive care units (ICU). Several meta-analysis studies have been published underlining its efficacy and significance in the reduction of infections in the critically ill patient, especially of ventilator-associated pneumonia (VAP) and bloodstream infections with consequent reductions of mortality by 20% [1–3].

Prevention of infections in the critically ill ICU patient by means of SDD is based on the observation that about 80% of the infections originating in ICUs are endogenous. This means that they are caused by microorganisms in the intestinal anal and oropharyngeal cavity of the patients, which are present on admission or acquired later on in the ICU. These infections can thus be either primary endogenous infections or infections that result after ICU-acquired secondary colonisation of the intestinal canal, i.e. secondary endogenous infections (see Chapter 2).

The principle of SDD is that by means of application of nonabsorbable antibiotics in the intestinal canal and oropharyngeal cavity potentially pathogenic microorganisms (PPM) are eliminated, thereby reducing the incidence of organ site infections, especially VAP. The endogenous anaerobic flora is preserved as a factor contributing to colonisation defence. The principles of this technique have been described many times, and it has in use in ICUs and in haemato-oncology since the late 1970s and since the early 1980s in the critically ill [4, 5].

Widespread use of this technique in the ICU is accepted with reluctance by traditional infectious disease specialists, microbiologists and opinion leaders in the field of critical care medicine. The major concern of those who reject the technique is the potential induction of antibiotic resistance that might result from the using of antibiotics in a prophylactic strategy.

However, basing a decision to withhold a life-saving strategy on opinion rather than on solid evidence is not in keeping in line with the principles of evidence-based medicine (EBM).

This review concerns the evaluation of SDD with particular reference to the onset of clinically relevant antimicrobial resistance.

Resistance in the ICU

An exponentially increasing number of studies report the problem of antimicrobial-resistant infections in critically ill patients resulting from the traditional approach to the control and treatment of infections in the ICU (Fig. 9.1).

This resistance problem is a major challenge to the intensivist [6]. Within the context of this study we focus on clinical aspects of antimicrobial resistance (AR) rather than upon the molecular-biological mechanisms of AR. In clinical practice the carriage of AR microorganisms develops in several stages.

First, it has been known for the last 30 years that critical illness is the most independent risk factor for acquisition and carriage of abnormal, often resistant, bacteria [7–9]. In healthy individuals such bacteria are easily cleared by internal mechanisms [10], whereas in critically ill, previously healthy, patient (e.g. a trauma patient) carriage will develop [4, 5].

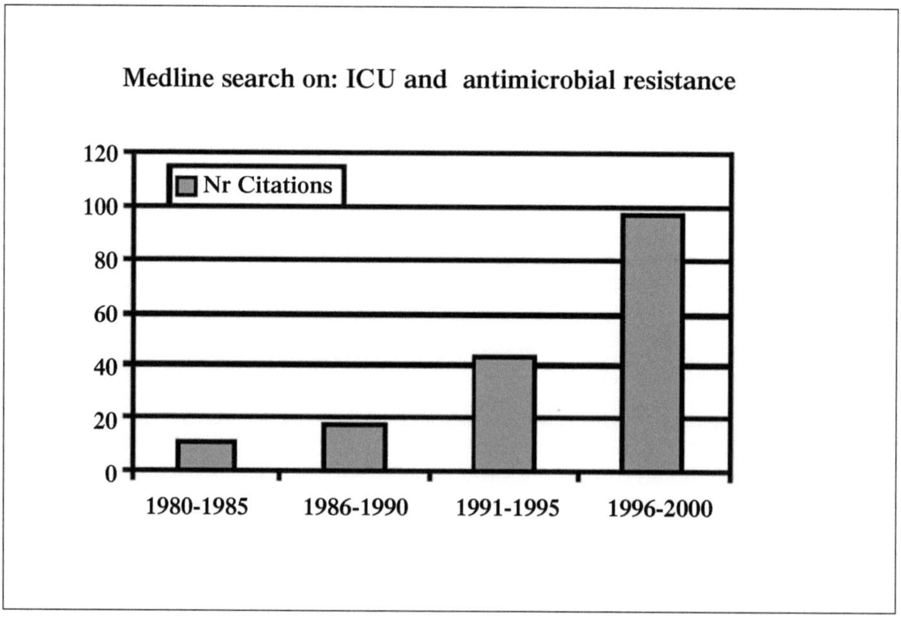

Fig. 9.1 Medline search on intensive care and microbial resistance

Secondly, for patients to become carriers of abnormal flora they must have been exposed to the abnormal microorganisms. Patients may carry abnormal flora on admission (import) or they may have normal flora on admission but subsequently acquire PPM in the ICU (acquisition).

Thirdly, following exposure critically ill patients may develop carriage, i.e. persistent presence of PPM in throat and gut. Healthy individuals do not become sustained carriers of potentially pathogenic microorganisms.

This abnormal carriage leads to the overgrowth of abnormal flora in the ICU patient. Overgrowth presents a serious problem in the ICU, for three reasons:

1. Overgrowth is required for carriage of resistant strains amongst the sensitive population.
2. Overgrowth is required for endogenous supercolonisation/infection of the individual patient.
3. Overgrowth of resistant microbes promotes dissemination throughout the ICU via the caregivers' hands.

Severity of Illness

Chronic and acute disease states are characterised by carriage of abnormal aerobic Gram-negative and Gram-positive flora. Patients with diabetes, alcoholism and COPD have been shown to carry abnormal microorganisms in 30% of cases [11–17]. Previously healthy trauma victims become carriers after the acute insult when they are treated in the ICU for their injuries [4].

The APACHE score assesses the combination of chronic health disability in combination with acute disturbances of the vital functions. Abnormal carrier status with aerobic Gram-negative bacteria intensifies with rising APACHE score. About 30% of patients with APACHE >15 become pathologically colonised. This colonisation significantly increases with APACHE >27, to affect over 50% of these patients [18].

Increasing SAPS is also associated with increased pathological carrier state of AGNB. It is evident that patients' illness causes the conversion of carriage of normal into abnormal flora.

Pre-ICU Antibiotics Use

Patients' endogenous reservoirs can be considered as the predominant source of abnormal microorganisms. From the intensivist's point of view, it is unlikely that short-stay patients who are in the ICU for less than four days will contribute to the spread of abnormal flora in the unit (no severe underlying disease). Patients with higher APACHE scores are responsible for the dissemination of abnormal flora. Faecal carriage is thought to be more important than nasal or oropharyngeal carriage, because more bacteria per gram of faeces than per millilitre of saliva are present.

Previous antibiotic use in critically ill patients prior to admission may already have contributed to abnormal carriage owing to acquired (by disease) and induced (by antibiotic use) disturbances of their resistance to colonisation. In a recent study we noted that 50% of the patients acutely admitted to the ICU had already been treated with systemic antibiotics prior to admission [19]. Epidemiological studies show that between 30% and 50% of resistant strains are imported into the ICU by patients requiring intensive treatment. This acquisition of abnormal flora almost always occurs in the first week of treatment in the ICU as the result of breaches of such barriers as indwelling catheters, of tracheotomies and of impaired resistance to colonisation as a consequence of systemic antibiotic treatment. The breakdown of colonisation resistance, i.e. the elimination of anaerobes from the intestinal canal, is associated with an increased risk of bloodstream infections (BSI) with enteral microorganisms.

Hand-washing will have no effect in patients who are already carrying AGNB, MRSA and VRE when they are admitted. This may explain the lack of studies demonstrating that relying on hygienic measures does not decrease the rate of VAP and septicaemia in the ICU [20].

Antibiotic resistance

The traditional approach to the control of resistance is based on:
1. Restrictive antibiotic use (limited prophylactic use; treatment of proven infections only)
2. Hygienic measures
3. Isolation.

In spite of stressing these aspects an increasing problem with AR is observed in ICUs (Fig. 9.1).

Intensivists are confronted with a majority of patients who have already been treated with antibiotics because of infections. Despite attempts to reduce their use, over 70% of patients staying over 3 days in an ICU will receive antibiotics [21]. Over 80% of VAP needing antibiotic treatment will develop within the first ten days in the ICU. This situation will inevitably lead to outbreaks of multi-resistant strains as the result of increased pathologic colonisation and overgrowth in the oropharynx and rectum. In the absence of surveillance cultures to identify carriage of PPM, parenteral antibiotics are necessarily used to control infections, but this contributes to further resistance problems because the carrier state is not treated (source remains). ICUs are then closed to new admissions until the final carriers are dead or have been discharged (thereby creating a new problem in the new ward). In The Netherlands, in the year 2000, over 10% of ICUs using this traditional approach to infection control had to be closed on occasion and subjected to intensive cleansing to control outbreaks of multi-resistant microorganisms [22]. This illustrates the fact that The Netherlands is not a “resistance-free country”, as it is usually perceived.

It is acknowledged that VAP is the most important infection in the ICU, being responsible for over 30% of infections in critically ill ICU patient.

The conventional way to control antibiotic usage in this condition is, first, to increase the specificity of the diagnosis of VAP by invasive methods, and secondly, to apply scheduled changes in antibiotic classes.

However, in a French study comparing protected specimen brush versus tracheal aspirate for diagnosis of VAP the resistance problem was identical: 61.3% versus 59.8%, despite a significant reduction in the use of antibiotics in the protected specimen brush group [23]. A recent work has shown no impact of the use of invasive diagnostic tools, such as protected specimen brush rather than tracheal aspirate in the diagnosis, duration of mechanical ventilation, number of days in the ICU and mortality, as sampling methods for diagnostic specimen [24].

Changing antimicrobial classes may be temporarily effective. However, after 4–6 weeks intestinal overgrowth of multi-resistant strains will again lead to carriage of multi-resistant strains and to subsequent organ site infections [25].

In spite of these measures the success rate of the treatment of nosocomial pneumonia, usually VAP, in the ICU remains disappointingly low, with microbiological cure rates between 80-90% and onset of resistance [26–28].

Isolation as infection prevention does not prevent infections of endogenous origin but does delay the onset of exogenous infections [29].

The SDD Approach

As outlined above, the underlying concept is that ill patients will develop overgrowth of abnormal flora, which is exacerbated by the administration of systemic antibiotics that leave normal flora undisturbed. From this concept it follows that the SDD approach has four components:

1. Twice-weekly microbiological surveillance of throat and gut flora;
2. Eradication of overgrowth with appropriate topical nonabsorbable antimicrobials;
3. Use of pre-1980s systemic antimicrobial agents that respect the ecology for empirical treatment when necessary, for a maximum period of 5 days;
4. High standards of hygiene to control transmission of PPM.

The hypothesis that control of overgrowth of PPM by SDD will control resistance has been tested in experimental, paediatric and adult settings [30–32].

The safety of SDD relies on the fact that resistance is not emerging against the SDD antimicrobials in long-term use. A recent meta-analysis [1] examining 33 randomised SDD trials involving 5,727 patients confirmed the virtual absence of any reported resistance over a period of more than ten years

(1987–1997) and of subsequent superinfections and/or epidemics attributable to multi-resistant strains. Antimicrobial resistance, being a long-term issue, has been evaluated in eleven SDD studies over periods varying between two and nine years. These studies show no evidence of antimicrobial resistance [33–43].

Two studies evaluating the emergence of resistant microorganisms after discontinuation of SDD have failed to show any negative effect [43, 44]. Recently, Silvestri et al. analysed resistance data from the fifty-six RCTs and ten meta-analyses, demonstrating that the data do not provide any evidence for a link between SDD and the emergence of antimicrobial resistance [45].

Aerobic Gram-negative bacilli

There are two RCTs available with the primary end-point of antimicrobial resistance amongst AGNB [46,47]. In the largest individual RCT involving about 1,000 patients, there were significantly fewer patients who carried AGNB resistant to tobramycin, imipenem, or ciprofloxacin amongst the patients receiving SDD than in the control group. Addition of enteral antimicrobials to the parenteral antibiotics controlled an outbreak attributable to extended-spectrum beta-lactamase (ESBL) producing *Klebsiella* spp. in a Parisian ICU. The carriage rate in the SDD group was 1%, whilst in the control group was 20%. There were no patients with infections in the SDD group, whilst 9% of the patients who only received the enteral agent developed infections with ESBL producing *Klebsiella*. Most ICU patients have microbial overgrowth, and gut overgrowth has been shown to guarantee increased spontaneous mutation, leading to polyclonality and antimicrobial resistance [48]. The enteral antimicrobials polymyxin and tobramycin eradicate and/or prevent gut overgrowth caused by AGNB and may explain the absence of antimicrobial resistance among AGNB.

The efficacy of the SDD regimen in controlling outbreaks of infection with multi-resistant Gram-negative bacteria has been reported several times [47–50]. This topic is discussed in detail in Chapter 11.

Extended-spectrum beta-lactamase

The emergence of ESBL-producing microorganisms due to SDD has not been described. Recently it was suggested that ESBL might be a problem in ICUs in which SDD is used [51]. This topic is discussed in more detail in Chapter 11.

Methicillin-resistant **Staphylococcus aureus**

SDD is not designed to deal with MRSA. Of the fifty-six RCTs, seven were undertaken in units with endemic MRSA [52–58]. These seven RCTs involving about 2,000 patients show a trend towards higher MRSA infection rates amongst patients receiving PTA. In the case of MRSA endemicity, enteral vancomycin should be added to PTA [59]. Enteral vancomycin guarantees high faecal levels varying between 3,000 and 24,000 μg/ml of faeces, whilst i.v. vancomycin 2 g results in homeopathic vancomycin levels (excreted via the bile) varying between 6 and 10 μg/ml faeces [60–62].

Vancomycin-resistant enterococci

There are two RCTs in which carriage and infection with vancomycin-resistant enterococci (VRE) are primary end-points. In both American RCTs carriage and infection rates were similar in both test and control groups [63, 64].

There are eight RCTs in which enteral vancomycin was added to the classic SDD (PTA) and VRE was not a problem [59, 65–71].

Recent animal work has demonstrated that parenteral antibiotics that disregard the gut ecology, rather than high doses of vancomycin, promote VRE [72,73].

The timely detection of VRE by twice-weekly surveillance cultures of the rectum has been suggested to be of value in the identification for patient at risk for infections caused by VRE. VRE infection occurs an average of eight days after acquired intestinal colonisation [74]. This study shows that for other than Gram-negative bacteria too, the intestinal carrier state is the crucial step in the pathogenesis of infections with such intestinal colonisers as VRE in the critically ill.

The spread of resistant microorganisms is influenced predominantly by the proportion of patients colonised. Reducing the proportion of colonised patients will automatically lower the chance of abnormal transmission of intestinal bacteria throughout the ICU. Acquisition of VRE is not prevented by the additional use of gowns in addition to gloves [75].

Conclusion

The ICU is the created epicentre of the resistance problem. The use of solely systemic antibiotics, whether restricted or not, maintains an abnormal population of bacteria amongst which resistance is encouraged. The eradication of the reservoir of abnormal bacteria located in the gut (i.e. colonisation pressure) by topical nonabsorbable antibiotics (i.e. decontamination) has been shown to be effective in significantly reducing morbidity, mortality and resistance. Perhaps the most intriguing experience in twenty years of clinical research into SDD is the observation that the addition of enteral to parenteral antimicrobials contributes to the control of antimicrobial resistance.

References

1. D'Amico R, Pifferi S, Leonetti C et al (1998) Effectiveness of antibiotic prophylaxis in critically ill adult patients: systematic review of randomised controlled trials. BMJ 316:1275-1285
2. Nathens AB, Marshall JC (1999) Selective decontamination of the digestive tract in surgical patients: a systematic review of the evidence. Arch Surg 134: 170-176
3. Heyland DK, Cook DJ, Jaeschke R et al (1994) Selective decontamination of the digestive tract. An overview. Chest 105:1221-1229
4. Stoutenbeek CP, van Saene HKF, Miranda DR et al (1987) The effect of oropharyngeal decontamination using topical non-absorbable antibiotics on the incidence of nosocomial respiratory infections in multiple trauma patients. J Trauma 27:357-364
5. Baxby D, van Saene HKF, Stoutenbeek CP et al (1996) Selective decontamination of the digestive tract: 13 years on, what it is and what it is not. Intensive Care Med 22:699-706
6. Fridkin SK, Gaynes RP (1999) Antimicrobial resistance in intensive care units. Clin Chest Med 20:303-316
7. Toltzis Ph, Yamashita T, Vilt L et al (1997) Colonization with antibiotic Gram-negative organisms in a paediatric intensive care unit. Crit Care Med 25:538-544
8. Garrouste-Orgeas M, Marie O, Rouveau M et al (1996) Secondary carriage with multi-resistant Acinetobacter baumannii and Klebsiella pneumoniae in an adult ICU population: relationship with nosocomial infections and mortality. J Hosp Infect 34: 279-289
9. Johanson WG, Pierce AK, Sanford JP (1969) Changing pharyngeal bacterial flora of hospitalized patients. Emergence of gram-negative bacilli. N Engl J Med 281:1137-1140
10. Van Saene HKF, Stoutenbeek CP, Geitz JN et al (1988) Effect of amoxycillin on 'colonisation resistance' in human volunteers. Microb Ecol Health Dis 1:169-177
11. Mobbs KJ, van Saene HKF, Sunderland D et al (1999) Oropharyngeal Gram-negative bacillary carriage. Chest 115:1570-1575
12. Mackowiak PA, Martin RM, Jones SR et al (1978) Pharyngeal colonisation by Gram-negative bacilli in aspiration prone persons. Arch Intern Med 138:1224-1227
13. Fuxench-Lopez Z, Ramirez-Ronda CH (1978) Pharyngeal flora in ambulatory alcoholic patients. Arch Intern Med 138:1815-1816
14. Mobbs KJ, van Saene HKF, Sunderland D et al (1999) Oropharyngeal Gram-negative bacillary carriage in chronic obstructive pulmonary disease: relation to severity of disease. Respir Med 93:540-545
15. Morris JG, Shay DK, Hebden JN et al (1995) Enterococci resistant to multiple antimicrobial agents, including vancomycin. Ann Intern Med 123:250-259
16. Coque TM, Tomayko JF, Ricke SC et al (1996) Vancomycin-resistant enterococci from nosocomial, community and animal sources in the United States. Antimicrob Agents Chemother 40:2605-2609
17. Pujol M, Pena C, Pallares R et al (1996) Nosocomial Staphylococcus aureus bacteremia among nasal carriers of methicillin-resistant and methicillin-susceptible strains. Am J Med 100:509-516
18. Sanchez-Garcia M, Cambronero-Galache JA, Lopez-Diaz J et al (1998) Effectiveness and costs of selective decontamination of the digestive tract in critically ill intubated patients. Am J Respir Crit Care Med 158:908-916
19. van der Voort PH, van der Hulst RW, Zandstra DF et al (2001) Suppression of Helicobacter pylori infection during intensive care stay: related to stress ulcer bleeding incidence? J Crit Care 16:182-187
20. Daschner FD, Frey P, Wolff G et al (1982) Nosocomial infections in intensive care wards: a multicenter prospective study. Intensive Care Med 8:5-9
21. Rangel-Frausto MS, Pittet D, Costigan M et al (1995) The natural history of the systemic inflammatory response syndrome (SIRS): a prospective study. JAMA 273:117-123
22. Source: Algemeen Nederlands Persbureau.

23. Fagon JY, Chastre J, Wolff M et al (2000) Invasive and non-invasive strategies for management of suspected ventilator-associated pneumonia. Ann Intern Med 132:621-630
24. Canadian Critical Care Trials Group; Heyland D, Dodek P, Muscedere J et al (2006) A randomized trial of diagnostic techniques for ventilator-associated pneumonia. N Engl J Med 355:2619-2630
25. de Man P, Verhoeven BA, Verbrugh HA et al (2000) An antibiotic policy to prevent emergence of resistant bacilli: Lancet 355:973-978
26. Wolff M (1998) Comparison of strategies using cefpirome and ceftazidime for empiric treatment of pneumonia in intensive care patients. The Cefpirome Pneumonia treatment group Antimicrob Agents Chemother 42:28-36
27. Brun-Buisson C, Sollet JP, Schweich H et al (1998) Treatment of ventilator-associated pneumonia with piperacillin-tazobactam/amikacin versus ceftazidime/amikacin: a multicenter, randomized controlled trial. VAP Study Group. Clin Infect Dis 26:346-354
28. Beaucaire G, Nicolas MH, Martin C (1999) Phare study. Comparative study of combined cefepime-amikacin versus ceftazidime combined with amikacin in the treatment of nosocomial pneumonias in ventilated patients. Multicenter group study. Ann Fr Anesth Reanim 18:186-195
29. Klein BS, Perloff WH, Maki DG (1989) Reduction of nosocomial infection during pediatric intensive care by protective isolation. N Engl J Med 320:1714-1721
30. van der Waaij D, van der Waaij JM (1985) Spread of multiresistant gram-negative bacilli among severely immuno-compromised mice during prophylactic treatment with different oral antimicrobial drugs. Prog Clin Biol Res 181:245-250
31. Baines PB, Taylor N, Sarginson RE et al. (2006) Emergence of antimicrobial resistance in a paediatric intensive care unit (PICU). Pediatr Crit Care Med Suppl 3rd World Congress, book of Abstracts, 165 FP16 Infectious Diseases.
32. de la Cal MA, Cerda E, Calderon M et al. Oral vancomycin in the control of MRSA outbreaks in ICU. In: van Saene HKF, Sganga G, Silvestri L (eds) Infection in the critically ill: an ongoing challenge. Springer-Verlag Italia, Milan 2001, pp 139-146
33. Hammond JMJ, Potgieter PD (1995) Long-term effects of selective decontamination on antimicrobial resistance. Crit Care Med 23:637-645
34. Stoutenbeek CP, van Saene HKF, Zandstra DF (1987) The effect of oral non-absorbable antibiotics on the emergence of resistant bacteria in patients in an intensive care unit. J Antimicrob Chemother 19:513-520
35. Lingnau W, Berger J, Javorsky F et al (1998) Changing bacterial ecology during a five-year period of selective intestinal decontamination. J Hosp Infect 39:195-206
36. van der Voort PHJ, van Roon EN, Kampinga GA et al (2004) A before-after study of multiresistance and cost of selective decontamination of the digestive tract. Infection 32:271-277
37. Viviani M, van Saene HK, Dezzoni R et al (2005) Control of imported and acquired methicillin-resistant Staphylococcus aureus (MRSA) in mechanically ventilated patients: a dose–response study of enteral vancomycin to reduce absolute carriage and infection. Anaesth Intensive Care 33:361-372
38. Sarginson RE, Taylor N, Reilly N et al (2004) Infection in prolonged pediatric critical illness: a prospective four-year study based on knowledge of the carrier state. Crit Care Med 32:839-842
39. Heininger A, Meyer E, Schwab F et al (2006) Effects of long-term routine use of selective digestive decontamination on antimicrobial resistance. Intensive Care Med 32:1569-1576
40. Leone M, Albanese J, Antonini F et al (2003) Long-term (6 year) effect of selective digestive decontamination on antimicrobial resistance in intensive care, multiple-trauma patients. Crit Care Med 31:2090-2095
41. De la Cal MA, Cerda E, van Saene HK et al (2004) Effectiveness and safety of enteral vancomycin to control endemicity of methicillin-resistant Staphylococcus aureus in a medical/surgical intensive care unit. J Hosp Infect 56:175-183
42. Cerda E, Abella A, de la Cal MA et al (2007) Enteral vancomycin controls methicillin-resist-

ant Staphylococcus aureus endemicity in an intensive care burn unit. A 9-year prospective study. Ann Surg 245:397-407
43. Tetteroo GWM, Wagenvoort JHT, Bruining HA (1994) Bacteriology of selective decontamination: efficacy and rebound colonization. J Antimicrob Chemother 34:529-544
44. Saunders N, Hammond JMJ, Potgieter PD et al (1994) Microbiological surveillance during selective decontamination of the digestive tract (SDD). J Antimicrob Chemother 34:529-544
45. Silvestri L, van Saene HK (2006) Selective decontamination of the digestive tract does not increase resistance in critically ill patients: evidence from randomized controlled trials. Crit Care Med 34:2027-2029
46. de Jonge E, Schultz MJ, Spanjaard L et al (2003) Effects of selective decontamination of digestive tract on mortality and acquisition of resistant bacteria in intensive care: a randomised controlled trial. Lancet 362(9389):1011-1016
47. Brun-Buisson C, Legrand P, Rauss A et al (1989) Intestinal decontamination for control of nosocomial multi-resistant –gram-negative bacilli. Ann Intern Med 110:873-881
48. Damjanovic V, van Saene HK (2005) Microbial mutation as a source of polyclonality in the gut of the critically ill. J Hosp Infect 59:374-375
49. Taylor ME, Oppenheim BA (1991) Selective decontamination of the gastrointestinal tract as an infection control measure. J Hosp Infect 71:271-278
50. Agusti C, Pujol M, Argerich MJ et al (2002) Short-term effect of the application of selective decontamination of the digestive tract on different body site reservoir ICU patients colonized by multi-resistant Acinetobacter baumannii. J Antimicrob Chemother 49:205-208
51. Al Naiemi N, Heddema ER, Bart A et al (2006) Emergence of multidrug-resistant Gram-negative bacteria during selective decontamination of the digestive tract on an intensive care unit. J Antimicrob Chemother 58:853-856
52. Gastinne H, Wolff M, Delatour F et al (1992) A controlled trial in intensive care units of selective decontamination of the digestive tract with non-absorbable antibiotics. N Engl J Med 326:594-599
53. Hammond JM, Potgieter PD, Saunders GL et al (1992) Double-blind study of selective decontamination of the digestive tract in intensive care. Lancet 340:5-9
54. Ferrer M, Torres A, Gonzalez J et al (1994) Utility of selective digestive decontamination in mechanically ventilated patients. Ann Intern Med 120:389-395
55. Wiener J, Itokazu G, Nathan C et al (1995) A randomized, double-blind, placebo controlled trial of selective digestive decontamination in a medical, surgical intensive care unit. Clin Infect Dis 20:861-867
56. Lingnau W, Berger J, Javorsky F et al (1997) Selective intestinal decontamination in multiple trauma patients: prospective, controlled trial. J Trauma 42:687-694
57. Verwaest C, Verhaegen J, Ferdinande P et al (1997) Randomized controlled trial of selective digestive decontamination in 600 mechanically ventilated patients in a multi-disciplinary intensive care unit. Crit Care Med 25:63-71
58. De la Cal MA, Cerda E, Garcia-Hierro P et al (2005) Survival benefit in critically ill burned patients receiving selective decontamination of the digestive tract: a randomized, placebo-controlled, double-blind trial. Ann Surg 241:424-430
59. Silvestri L, van Saene HK, Milanese M et al (2004) Prevention of MRSA pneumonia by oral vancomycin decontamination: a randomised trial. Eur Respir J 23:921-926
60. Geraci JE, Heilman FR, Nichols DR et al (1956) Some laboratory and clinical experiences with a new antibiotic, vancomycin. Mayo Clin Proc 31:564-582
61. Currie BP, Lemos-Filho L (2004) Evidence for biliary excretion of vancomycin into stool during intravenous therapy: potential implications for rectal colonization with vancomycin-resistant enterococci. Antimicrob Agents Chemother 48:4427-4429
62. Tedesco F, Markham R, Gurwith M et al (1978) Oral vancomycin for antibiotic-associated pseudomembranous colitis. Lancet II/8083:226-228
63. Arnow PM, Carandang GC, Zabner R et al (1996) Randomized controlled trial of selective bowel decontamination for prevention of infections following liver transplantation. Clin Infect Dis 22:997-1003

64. Hellinger WC, Yao JD, Alvarez S et al (2002) A randomized, prospective, double-blinded evaluation of selective bowel decontamination in liver transplantation. Transplantation 73:1904-1909
65. Bergmans DC, Bonten MJ, Gaillard CA et al (2001) Prevention of ventilator-associated pneumonia by oral decontamination: a prospective, randomized, double-blind, placebo-controlled study. Am J Respir Crit Care Med 164:382-388
66. Gaussorgues P, Salord F, Sirodot M et al (1991) Efficacité de la décontamination digestive sur la survenue des bactériémies nosocomiales chez les patients sous ventilation méchanique et recevant des betamimétiques. Réanimation Soins Intensifs Médecin d'Urgence 7:169-174
67. Korinek AM, Laisne MJ, Nicolas MH et al (1993) Selective decontamination of the digestive tract in neurosurgical intensive care unit patients: a double-blind, randomized, placebo-controlled study. Crit Care Med 21:1466-1473
68. Krueger WA, Lenhart FP, Neeser G et al (2002) Influence of combined intravenous and topical antibiotic prophylaxis on the incidence of infections, organ dysfunctions, and mortality in critically ill surgical patients: a prospective, stratified, randomized, double-blind, placebo-controlled clinical trial. Am J Respir Crit Care Med 166:1029-1037
69. Pugin J, Auckenthaler R, Lew DP et al (1991) Oropharyngeal decontamination decreases incidence of ventilator-associated pneumonia. A randomized, placebo-controlled, double-blind clinical trial. JAMA 265:2704-2710
70. Schardey HM, Joosten U, Finke U et al (1997) The prevention of anastomotic leakage after total gastrectomy with local decontamination. A prospective, randomized, double-blind, placebo-controlled multicenter trial. Ann Surg 225:172-180
71. Sanchez M, Mir N, Canton R, Luque R et al (1997) The effect of topical vancomycin on acquisition, carriage and infection with methicillin-resistant Staphylococcus aureus in critically ill patients. A double-blind, randomised, placebo-controlled study. 37th ICAAC, 1997, Toronto, Canada, Abstract J-119, p. 310
72. Stiefel U, Paterson DL, Pultz NJ et al (2004) Effect of the increasing use of piperacillin/tazobactam on the incidence of vancomycin-resistant enterococci in four academic medical centers. Infect Control Hosp Epidemiol 25:380-383
73. Salgado CD, Gianetta ET, Farr BM (2004) Failure to develop vancomycin-resistant enterococci in San Francisco Bay area hospitals during 1994 to 1998. Infect Control Hosp Epidemiol 25:413-417
74. Hendrix CW, Hammond JMJ, Swoboda SM et al (2001) Surveillance strategies and impact of vancomycin-resistant enterococcal colonisation and infection in critically ill patients. Ann Surg 233:259-265
75. Slaughter S, Hayden MK, Nathan C et al (1996) A comparison of the effect of universal use of gloves and gowns with that of glove alone on acquisition of vancomycin resistant enterococci in a medical intensive care unit. Ann Intern Med 125:448-456

Chapter 10
The Costs of SDD

Peter H.J. van der Voort

Introduction

In recent years, the cost of intensive care treatment has become increasingly important to managers and medical professionals. In fact, every treatment could be discussed in the context of a cost–benefit analysis. At present, most hospitals have a committee that studies the need for all newly introduced medications and facilities. A cost analysis is usually performed. If SDD is introduced in a hospital, the medical staff and managers may be confronted with the question of its cost and benefits. The purpose of this chapter is to review the current literature relating to the cost of SDD.

The Problems of Cost Analysis

The costs involved in intensive care treatment are difficult to analyse. Many different factors can play a part. An increase in costs may easily be counteracted by cost reductions in other aspects of intensive care treatment. In addition, the way an intensive care unit is organised determines the overhead costs. The costs of a treatment may vary between hospitals because their negotiations with a manufacturer have resulted in different prices for the same products. This is particularly true for intravenous antibiotics. In addition, legislation and organisation at national level will probably also affect the cost of intensive care.

Costs

Costs can be divided in different categories [1]. Direct costs are costs of goods, services and other resources that are consumed in the provision of a health intervention and can be medical or nonmedical [1]. In this category, patient care is

P.H.J. van der Voort, H.K.F. van Saene (eds.) *Selective Digestive Tract Decontamination in Intensive Care Medicine.* © Springer 2008

the cost-object. Indirect costs (overhead costs) are the costs of resources that are being generated by multiple cost-objects. The distinction between direct and indirect costs is sometimes difficult. A distinction can also be made between fixed and variable costs. Fixed costs cannot be determined by ICU production. On the other hand, variable costs are related to ICU production. The severity of disease is related to the variable costs. Marginal costs are those costs that are the result of an increase of production by one unit.

Two methods of calculating total costs are the 'top-down' and 'bottom-up' methods. In the top-down method the costs are calculated from the overall organisation towards a smaller unit (e.g. one patient). This method is a retrospective approach. The bottom-up approach calculates the costs (prospectively) starting from the individual patient.

Cost Analysis of SDD

A cost analysis of SDD may include direct and variable costs resulting from the implementation of SDD as part of the standard intensive care treatment and also the effects of SDD on the standard intensive care treatment. These effects can include, for instance, a reduced frequency of bronchoscopy and bronchoalveolar lavage (BAL) because of the lower incidence of ventilator-associated pneumonia. Overhead costs are less important. The most important variable costs are the costs of antibiotics. These costs can be divided into costs of the local, topical antibiotics (those applied in the oropharynx and through the gastric tube) and the parenteral, systemic antibiotics. Systemic, i.v., antibiotics can be given for the first four days of ICU stay, when they are intended to treat colonisation and early infection (usually a third-generation cephalosporin, most often cefotaxime), or later in the intensive care stay for the treatment of newly acquired infection. As the topical and early systemic antibiotics are meant as a strategy to prevent infection, a reduction of infections during the total intensive care stay and, as a consequence, a reduction in total antibiotic use can be expected. This hypothesis was recently confirmed in a prospective trial [2]. In this kind of cost analysis one needs to know the number of vials used, the kind of antibiotic and the price that the local pharmacist pays to the manufacturer. The price of the i.v. antibiotics is heavily dependent on the local pharmacy and can vary widely between hospitals.

Literature

The available literature can be divided into three groups of studies: (1) Oral decontamination without gastrointestinal decontamination; (2) oral and gastrointestinal decontamination without i.v. antibiotics; (3) the complete SDD regimen with oral and gastrointestinal decontamination and a 3- to 4-day course of i.v. antibiotics.

Ad 1. The study by Abele [3] was a small study of patients selected for SDD, who received no topical administration of SDD suspension in the gastrointestinal tract. Only oral paste was applied topically, and cefotaxime was administered i.v. for three days. Overall, antibiotic use with the SDD regimen was cheaper. Other costs were not analysed.

Ad 2. Other studies with oral and gastrointestinal decontamination but without systemic antibiotics over the first few days show variable outcomes. Some show a decrease in costs [4–8], some find higher costs [9–12], and one study found similar costs with or without SDD [13].

Ad 3. The studies that analysed costs of the complete SDD regimen, consisting of cefotaxime i.v. in addition to oral and gastric decontamination, are those conducted by Stoutenbeek [14], Schardey [15], de Jonge [2] and van der Voort [16]. These studies all showed a reduction in costs, even though the costs were analysed in different ways in all the studies.

Two studies using quinolones as the standard i.v. antibiotic showed higher costs [17, 18]. Two studies in which other cephalosporins were used showed lower or unchanged costs of antibiotics [19, 20].

Although it is difficult to compare the studies, it is reasonable to conclude that the complete regimen (oral plus gastrointestinal decontamination plus i.v. cephalosporin) brings about the most consistent cost reduction.

The available studies can be analysed for specific groups of patients, e.g. liver transplant patients, trauma patients and gastrectomy patients. Three studies have discussed the costs of SDD for liver transplant patients [11–13, 20]. The studies published by van Enckevort [11] and Zwaveling [12] were performed in the same patients. In one study [20] i.v. antibiotics (second-generation cephalosporin) were used, and in the other two studies no intravenous antibiotics were used. Two studies showed similar costs whether SDD was used or not [13, 20], whilst in the other study [11, 12] the costs were also similar except that in the SDD group costs for SDD medication were added, leading to an increase in total costs. One of the problems of this study [11, 12] is that the patients in the SDD group received norfloxacin and lozenges containing polymyxin, tobramycin and amphotericin for a mean of 4 months, which contributes to high costs.

In the case of trauma patients, cost was analysed in only one study using the complete SDD regimen [14]. Two other studies in this patient population did not use i.v. antibiotics [4, 8]. The study using the complete regimen showed a reduction in costs, while the other two studies did not.

The one study in patients undergoing gastrectomy showed a decrease in costs with SDD [15]. In this study the patients received the complete SDD regimen.

Other Organisations

The Agency for Healthcare Research and Quality in the USA has written guidelines on patient safety practice and targets [21]. In Chapter 17 of these guidelines the prevention of ventilator-associated pneumonia is addressed, and section 17.3 discusses selective digestive tract decontamination. Concerning costs, the following analysis of available trials is made: *'The cost of implementing SDD appears minimal in most trials, but there have been no in depth reviews of the subject. Several trials have found that patients receiving SDD had lower total antibiotic costs. Overall hospital costs also may be lower, mediated through the decreased rate of VAP.'* And: *'SDD is a relatively non-invasive intervention and the additional financial cost is minimal.'*

Discussion

There have been no studies with the primary end-point of cost-effectiveness of SDD. In a limited number of studies the costs of SDD have been studied as a secondary end-point. These studies have analysed several kinds of costs, which were not equally well defined. Table 10.1 shows the main results of these studies. The conclusions of the studies are inconsistent owing to differences in study design and variation in costs definition and in local influences. For instance, the costs of topical therapy vary widely from $4 [19], through $5.25 [4] and $17 [5] to $70 [6] per day. The use of systemically active, i.v.-administered antibiotics varies widely between hospitals ($20–70/day) and largely determines the overall costs. It is of the utmost importance that the local pharmacy buys the antibiotics for the lowest possible price. The oral paste and gastrointestinal suspension are not available commercially. When preparing these items, the pharmacist should use the cheapest available ingredients. Use of the i.v. formulation of tobramycin in the paste and suspension greatly increases the costs of these. The costs for cephotaxime, in our experience, can be 4 or 5 times as high in one hospital as in another. This variation can have a huge influence on the calculated costs and makes it difficult to compare studies. Specific information on the costs per dose is usually not provided in the available studies.

The costs for the microbiological laboratory have received relatively limited attention [11, 16]. The total number of cultures will increase owing to the surveillance cultures, although this is not true for ICUs performing surveillance cultures without SDD. However, under the SDD regimen, the cultures will usually show Gram-positive flora, which does not need further analysis in throat and rectal swaps. Cultures of organ sites (trachea, urine, abdominal cavity, etc.) need determination of Gram-positive flora for the detection of *Staphylococcus aureus*, coagulase-negative rods and amoxicillin-resistant enterococci, as these bacteria need specific attention and, possibly, treatment. Only limited detection of resistance is needed. Resistance for cephalosporins, amoxicillin and vancomycin is enough to know. Therefore, the way culture samples should be analysed by the microbiological laboratory varies depending on sample site and microorganism. As a result, it does not make sense to have a standard price for a culture. Calculating the exact costs for the microbiological laboratory is time consuming

Table 10.1 Main results obtained in terms of cost of SDD in studies in which this was considered (Multiple Organ Dysfunction Syndrome, MODS)

First author [ref.]	Population	Study type	Country	Systemic antibiotics	Topical antibiotics	Antibiotic costs	Costs of cultures	Other costs	Length of stay in ICU	Costs per survivor	Conclusion
Abele-Horn 1997 [3]	MODS: 30 P; 58 SDD	RCT	D	Cefotaxime	PTA (oral only)	SOD lower	NA	NA	Decrease in SDD group	NA	Overall decrease by SOD
Rocha 1992 [17]	MODS: 47 P; 54 SDD	RCT	Sp	None	PTA	SDD lower	NA	NA	Unchanged	26% lower in SDD group	Overall decrease by SDD
Gastinne 1992 [10]	MODS; 225 P, 220 SDD	RCT	Fr	None	PTA	SDD higher	NA	NA	NA	NA	Increase in costs by SDD
Rolando 1993 [20]	Liver transplantation	RCT	UK	Cefuroxime	PTA	Unchanged	NA	NA	Unchanged	NA	Costs the same
Sanchez 1998 [19]	MODS; 140 P, 131 SDD	RCT	Sp	Ceftriaxon	PGA	SDD lower	Fixed price per culture	All ICU costs lower in SDD group	Unchanged	21% lower in SDD group	Overall decrease by SDD
Verwaest 1997 [17]	Surgical; 185 C; 193 OA; 200 PTA	RCT	Be	Ofloxacin or Cefotaxime	OA or PTA	Unchanged	NA	NA	Increase in SDD group	NA	Total costs per patient higher by SDD
Quinio 1996 [4]	Trauma	RCT	Fr	None	PGA	SDD lower	NA	NA	NA	NA	Antibiotic costs lower by SDD
Langlois 1994 [8]	Trauma; 47 SDD; 50 P	RCT	Fr	None	PGA	SDD lower	NA	NA	Unchanged	NA	Antibiotics costs lower by SDD
Wiener 1995 [9]	MODS; 31 C; 30 SDD	RCT	USA	None	PGN	SDD higher	NA	NA	Unchanged	NA	Antibiotic costs higher by SDD
Stoutenbeek 1996 [14]	Trauma; 30 SDD; 29 P	RCT	NL	Cefotaxime	PTA	SDD lower	NA	Lower transfusion costs	Decrease in SDD group	33% reduced in SDD group	Total costs lower by SDD
Lignau 1997 [18]	Trauma; 148 P; 162 SDD	RCT	Au	Ciproxin	PTA en PCA	SDD higher	NA	NA	NA	NA	Antibiotic costs higher by SDD
Korinek 1993 [6]	Neurosurgical; 63 SDD; 60 P	RCT	Fr	None	PTA	SDD lower	NA	NA	Unchanged	Lower in SDD group	Total costs lower by SDD
Nieuwenhoven [5]	MODS; 120 C; 61 SDD	RCT	NL	None	(oral only)	Control higher	Control higher	Unchanged	Unchanged	Reduced in SOD group	Total costs lower by SOD
Schardey 1997 [15]	Gastrectomy; 103 C; 90 SDD	RCT	Ge	Cefotaxime	PTA + vancomycin	SDD lower	NA	Re-operation	Reduced by SDD	NA	19% overall cost reduction
Hellinger 2002 [13]	Liver transplant	RCT	USA	None	PGN	NA	NA	Total medical care	Same	NA	Overall costs the same in both groups
De Jonge [2]	MODS; 468 P; 466 SDD	RCT	NL	Cefotaxime	PTA	SDD lower	NA	NA	NA	NA	Antibiotic costs 11% lower by SDD
V Enckevort/Zwaveling [11, 12]	Liver transplant; 29 P; 29 SDD	RCT	NL	None	PTA	?	SDD higher	Unchanged	Unchanged	NA	
Van der Voort 2004 [16]	MODS	Observational	NL	Cefotaxime	PTA	SDD higher	SDD higher	Reduction by SDD	Reduced by SDD	NA	Overall costs the same in both groups

RCT= Randomized Controlled Trial; PTA = Polymyxin, Tobramycin, Amphotericin B; PGA = Polymyxin, Gentomycin, Amphotericin B; PGN = Polymyxin, Gentomycin, Neomycin; OA = Ofloxacin, Amphotericin B; NA = Not Available; SOD = Selective Oral Decontamination

and has been undertaken in only two studies [11, 16]. The number of cultures was shown to double when SDD was begun. However, half of the cultures were surveillance cultures from throat or rectum, which involved only a limited workload because of Gram-positive flora that did not need further analysis. Overall, the mean price per culture may be around $15 for the surveillance cultures.

In some studies, the length of stay in the ICU is shortened during SDD, leading to a reduction in ICU treatment costs (variable direct costs). A VAP costs around 5 extra days of ICU treatment and a BSI, around ten extra ICU days. Prevention of these infections can substantially decrease length of stay and thus reduce the costs per patient. This can compensate for an increase in costs of any other SDD effect. However, length of stay can be highly variable between ICUs owing to organisational factors such as the presence of intensivists and step-down facilities, but also case mix.

The total costs can be divided by the number of survivors to produce cost per survivor. This produces a link between cost and effect. However, in smaller studies with a nonsignificant survival benefit for SDD owing to lack of power it is not possible to analyse costs in this way.

Conclusion

A reasonable number of studies have addressed the question of costs of SDD as against a standard antimicrobial regimen. However, none of the available studies that have addressed the cost of SDD has been designed to analyse its cost as a primary end-point. The method of cost analysis differs widely between studies and, as a result the conclusions concerning costs of SDD vary. Despite these drawbacks, all studies analysing the costs when the complete and 'original' SDD regimen is used (oral plus gastrointestinal decontamination and a short course of i.v. cefotaxime) show a reduction in antimicrobial or total costs. Incomplete or modified SDD regimens usually show a reduction in costs, but some studies show an increase in antibiotic costs.

References

1. Jegers M, Edbrooke DL, Hibbert CL et al (2002) Definitions and methods of cost assessment: an intensivist's guide. Intensive Care Med 28:680-685
2. De Jonge E, Schulz MJ, Spanjaart L et al (2003) Effects of Selective Decontamination of the Digestive tract on mortality and acquisition of resistant bacteria in intensive care: a randomised controlled trial. Lancet 362:1011-1016
3. Abele-Horn M, Dauber A, Bauernfeind A et al (1997) Decrease in nosocomial pneumonia in ventilated patients by selective oropharyngeal decontamination (SOD). Intensive Care Med 23:187-195
4. Quinio B, Albanese J, Bues-Charbit M et al (1996) Selective decontamination if the digestive tract in multiple trauma. Chest 109:765-772

5. Van Nieuwenhoven CA, Buskens E, Bergmans DC, Van Tiel F et al (2004) Oral decontamination is cost-saving in the prevention of ventilator-associated Pneumonia in intensive care units. Crit Care Med 32:126-130
6. Korinek AM, Laisne MJ, Nicholas MH et al (1993) Selective decontamination of the digestive tract in neurosurgical intensive care unit patients. A double-blind, randomised, placebo-controlled study. Crit Care Med 21:1466-1473
7. Rocha LA, Martin MJ, Pita S, (1992) Prevention of nosocomial infection in critically ill patients by selective decontamination of the digestive tract: a randomised, double-blind, placebo-controlled study. Intensive Care Med 18:398-404
8. Langlois-Karaga A, Bues-Charbit M, Davignon A et al (1995) Selective digestive decontamination in multiple trauma patients: cost and efficacy. Pharm World Sci 17:12-16
9. Wiener J, Itokazu G, Nathan C (1995) A randomized, double-blind, placebo-controlled trial of selective digestive decontamination in a medical-surgical intensive care unit. Clin Infect Dis 20:861-867
10. Gastinne H, Wolff M, Delatour F et al (1992) A controlled trial in intensive care units of selective decontamination of the digestive tract with non-absorbable antibiotics. N. Engl J Med 326:594-599
11. Van Enckevort PJ, Zwaveling JH, Bottema JT et al (2001) Cost effectiveness of selective decontamination of the digestive tract in liver transplant patients. Pharmacoeconomics 19:523-530
12. Zwaveling JH, Maring JK, Klompmaker IJ et al (2002) Selective decontamination of the digestive tract to prevent postoperative infection: A randomized placebo-controlled trial in liver transplant patients. Crit Care Med 30:1204-1209
13. Hellinger WC, Yao JD, Alvarez S et al (2002) A randomised, prospective, double-blind evaluation of selective bowel decontamination in liver transplantation. Transplantation 73:1904-1909
14. Stoutenbeek CP, van Saene HKF, Zandstra DF (1996) Prevention of multiple organ system failure by selective decontamination of the digestive tract in multiple trauma patients. In: Faist EBAE, Baue AE, Schildberg FW(eds) The immune consequences of trauma, shock and sepsis–mechanisms and therapeutic approaches.. Lengerich: Pabst Science Publishers, pp 1055-1066
15. Schardey HM, Joosten U, Finke U et al (1997) Kostensenkung durch Dekontamination zur Prävention der Nahtinsuffizienz nach Gastrectomie. Chirurg 68:416-424
16. van der Voort PHJ, van Roon EN, Kampinga GA et al (2004) A before–after study of multi-resistance and cost of selective decontamination of the digestive tract. Infection 32:271-277
17. Verwaest C, Verhaegen J, Ferdinande P et al (1997) Randomized controlled trial of selective digestive decontamination in 600 mechanically ventilated patients in a multidisciplinary intensive care unit. Crit Care Med 25:63-71
18. Lingnau W, Berger J, Javorsky F et al (1997) Selective intestinal decontamination in multiple trauma patients: prospective, controlled trial. J Trauma 42:687-693
19. Sanchez Garcia M, Cambronero Galache A, Lopez Diaz J et al (1998) Effectiveness and cost of selective decontamination of the digestive tract in critically ill intubated patients. Am J Respir Crit Care Med 158:908-916
20. Rolando N, Gimson A, Wade J et al (1993) Prospective controlled trial of selective parenteral and enteral antimicrobial regimen in fulminant liver failure. Hepatology 17:196-201
21. Making health care safer: a critical analysis of patient safety practices 2001. www.ahrq.gov/clinic/ptsafety

Chapter 11
SDD for the Prevention and Control of Outbreaks

Hans I. van der Spoel and Rik T. Gerritsen

Introduction

Outbreaks of infection with multi-resistant microorganisms are an increasing problem in intensive care units. Such outbreaks lead to increased mortality, longer duration of stay, higher costs and reduced availability of ICU beds [1, 2]. Many guidelines advocate strict adherence to hygiene measures, patient isolation and antibiotic restriction, but in spite of good and sometimes even supervised adherence to these measures, they often fail to contain the outbreak [3, 4]. An outbreak sometimes results in the temporary closure of the ICU [5, 6]. The normal measures taken to control an outbreak cause a lot of extra work for the medical and nursing staff. It is therefore important to control outbreaks as soon as possible when they occur, and even more important to apply measures to prevent outbreaks.

In this chapter, we will address the background and patterns of microbiology that lead to an outbreak. In addition, the different multi-resistant organisms involved will be discussed, with the emphasis on the need to apply a broader concept of infection control, including the use of surveillance cultures and methods of controlling and eliminating colonisation, which otherwise leads to subsequent infection. We will not discuss the role of molecular techniques and polyclonicity, as this is beyond the scope of this book [7, 8].

What Is an Outbreak?

An outbreak in ICU terms is an event in which two patients or more develop an *infection* or *colonisation* caused by the same, in general multi-resistant, potentially pathogenic microorganism (PPM) following transmission in an enclosed environment within a period of two weeks. *Endemicity* is an ongoing outbreak that is not controlled by any manoeuvre. An outbreak of infection should be distinguished from an outbreak of carriage. From a prevention point of view, an outbreak of carriage of multi-resistant PPM, e.g. MRSA, multi-resistant *Pseudomonas* or *Acinetobacter*, requires treatment because carriage will lead to infection and/or transmission [9, 10]. The detection of the carrier state of multi-resistant PPM by means of regular surveillance cultures of throat and rectum is indispensable in order to monitor the flora in the intensive care unit, so that emerging resistance can be detected in an early phase [11, 12] (see also Chapter 4).

Pathogenesis

There are three major elements in the development of an outbreak: source, transmission and susceptible host.

Source. The source is generally a critically ill patient with a minimum of three days of mechanical ventilation. Only in a minority of outbreaks (30%), it is a patient who is already carrying a multi-resistant microorganism on admission to the ICU [7]. Most ICU interventions promote overgrowth, which is defined as equal to or more than 10^5 multi-resistant bacteria per gram of faeces. Opiates, pharmaceutical stress ulcer prophylaxis and broad-spectrum antibiotics invariably lead to a carrier state owing to overgrowth. Opiates impair gut motility, while H_2-antagonists and proton pump inhibitors reduce the gastric barrier by increasing pH above 4. Broad-spectrum antimicrobials promote overgrowth via suppression of the normal indigenous flora, which is required to control abnormal flora. High concentrations of aerobic Gram-negative bacteria (AGNB) invariably contain resistant mutants, even if in very low counts. Most i.v.-administered antimicrobials are excreted via the bile into the faeces, eliminating the sensitive bacteria and selecting resistant mutants [13]. Selective antimicrobial pressure is thought to be responsible for 30% of resistant strains in the unit; 30% of the resistant strains are imported by patients carrying multi-resistant microorganisms on admission; and the remaining 40% are transmitted.

Transmission. Transmission of resistant PPM is virtually impossible to control in a unit in which there are patients with overgrowth [14, 15]. Washing a patient or changing the diaper of a baby with gut overgrowth of 10^9 bacteria leads to contamination of the hands of carers with up to 10^6 per square centimetre of finger surface. Rigid hand washing using 0.5% chlorhexidine in 70% alcohol reduces hand contamination at the most by 10^4 bacteria, still leaving 100 or more bacterial cells per square centimetre of finger surface present for transmission to other patients [16]. These quantitative data explain why hand-washing can reduce transmission but not completely abolish it [16, 17]. Obviously, transmission can occur not only via the hands of healthcare workers, but also by way of contaminated equipment, e.g. endoscopes, humidifiers, etc. Transmission is directly correlated with overall bacterial load [18]. Reducing the number of colonised patients with SDD will also reduce the size of the major source available for cross-contamination, be it through direct or through indirect transmission [19–21]. At least one third of all nosocomial infections are thought to be due to cross-transmission [22].

Susceptible host. SDD reduces the need for systemic antibiotics, an important risk factor in the emergence of resistance [19, 23, 24]. Most of the time there will be at least two patients in the unit who are critically ill, to such a degree that they develop an infection following acquisition after admission to the unit. It is the degree of immune suppression and disruption of natural barriers that determines whether carriage leads to infection [25, 26].

Types of Outbreaks

There are two types of outbreaks in the ICU. An outbreak of secondary endogenous infection must be distinguished from an outbreak of exogenous infection. Secondary endogenous infection requires a phase of digestive tract colonisation before infection develops [25, 27]. In contrast, an outbreak via exogenous infection occurs without previous carriage; in other words, two or more patients with burn wounds might acquire MRSA wound infection or pneumonia without previous throat and gut carriage. Yeast outbreaks are generally secondary endogenous infections, as secondary carriage and subsequent massive overgrowth in the small intestine are required for translocation and fungaemia. *Staphylococcus aureus*, *Pseudomonas aeroginosa* and *Acinetobacter* are microorganisms that can cause either type of outbreak [28]. Often both secondary endogenous and exogenous infection are involved in an outbreak, and only surveillance cultures can distinguish between them [29]. If the source is an external one, such as contaminated equipment, removal of the source will end the outbreak. The duration of such an outbreak is usually limited, depending on the efficacy of searching for the common source. Contamination of the equipment occurs either via direct contamination (e.g. an endoscope not properly decontaminated after use in an infected patient) or through transmission via the hands of healthcare workers who are also caring for a critically ill patient with overgrowth, or via a telephone or keyboard from which a second healthcare worker transfers the microorganism [30]. In the last cases the equipment is only the vector, and in a minority of cases contamination of this equipment persists, making it a new source with no apparent connection to the original source, i.e. the patient. Outbreaks may last for months and sometimes years and result in increased mortality, morbidity and antibiotic use, reduced ICU capacity and increased costs [1, 2, 28, 29, 31].

The Role of SDD in Outbreak Control

The aim of SDD is to prevent the carrier state and to eradicate PPM, if present, impeding subsequent overgrowth. Colonisation and overgrowth are an independent risk factor for (1) endogenous infection in the individual patient, (2) the emergence of a resistant mutant and (3) transmission in the unit [26, 27]. Successful decontamination renders the critically ill patient who is a carrier of resistant AGNB, yeasts or MRSA on admission to the ICU, or becomes a carrier after acquiring one or more later on, free of these PPM following the enteral administration of polymyxin/tobramycin, amphotericin B and vancomycin. The use of enteral antibiotics has been demonstrated to reduce resistance [21, 32, 33]. Finally, keeping the number of colonised patients small by means of SDD reduces the major source for cross-contamination [19–21]. In addition, handwashing is more effective in a unit where long-stay patients are successfully decontaminated, as the level of contamination of the hands of carers is significantly reduced—without extra measures even strict adherence to hygiene measures alone will not stop an outbreak [14].

Aerobic Gram-Negative Bacilli

Even the most potent newer antimicrobials, including fluoroquinoles, extended-spectrum β-lactam antibiotics and carbapenems, fail to clear an abnormal carrier state of multi-resistant *Klebsiella*, *Pseudomonas* and *Acinetobacter*. One randomised controlled trial and one observational study are available in which SDD was used to control an outbreak of *Klebsiella* infection [9, 10]. In a French and an English ICU in which multi-resistant *Klebsiella* was endemic, reinforcement of traditional hygiene measures, including hand disinfection, failed to control the outbreaks. However, SDD did have an impact on both outbreaks. In the Paris trial, patients were randomised and given either enteral antibiotics or no antibiotics [9]. Faecal carriage of the outbreak strain was eliminated, and the outbreak was under control within eight weeks. In the Manchester ICU all patients received SDD, and the outbreak was stopped within three weeks [10]. SDD, albeit in a somewhat different composition (neomycin instead of tobramycin), reduced the incidence of nosocomial pneumonias during an outbreak with a multi-resistant *Pseudomonas aeruginosa* from 56% before to 5% after implementation [34].

An Example of An Outbreak with Multi-Resistant Acinetobacter

In our own 20-year experience of SDD in the twenty-bedded ICU (nine 2-bed and two isolation rooms plus an adjacent six-bed step-down unit) of the OLVG in Amsterdam, we have encountered only one small outbreak. In 1998, a multi-resistant *Acinetobacter baumannii* (MRAb, sensitive only to polymyxin, amikacin and imipenem-cilastin) was brought into the ICU by a patient with cardiac failure and pneumonia. Although it was known that he was a carrier of MRAb, this information was lost during his transfer to the ICU. He was initially admitted to a two-bed room in which the second bed was empty. After intubation it became known that the patient was a carrier of MRAb and he was transferred to an isolation room within one hour after admission. Specific treatment consisted of administration of imipenem-cilastin and amikacin i.v. polymyxin by nebuliser, and SDD given as normal. Consecutive surveillance cultures did not show MRAb, and specific therapy was discontinued and isolation lifted. Eventually the patient was transferred to the normal ward, where he died of progressive cardiac failure. The second patient was admitted to the same room as the index patient after the room had been empty for six days. Cultures on admission did not yield MRAb, but later MRAb was cultured from her sputum, while all other surveillance cultures remained negative. However, MRAb was cultured from the package of suction catheters in a drawer in the room. It is speculated that MRAb was introduced directly into her lungs during tracheal suction. In the following seven weeks, a further six patients acquired MRAb (Fig. 11.1). Table 11.1 shows the characteristics of the infected and noninfected patients during the outbreak. All patients were treated aggressively with topical antimicrobials, and in the case of an infection also with systemic therapy, while SDD was applied as usual. In all cases MRAb was eliminated, albeit in some cases not until after

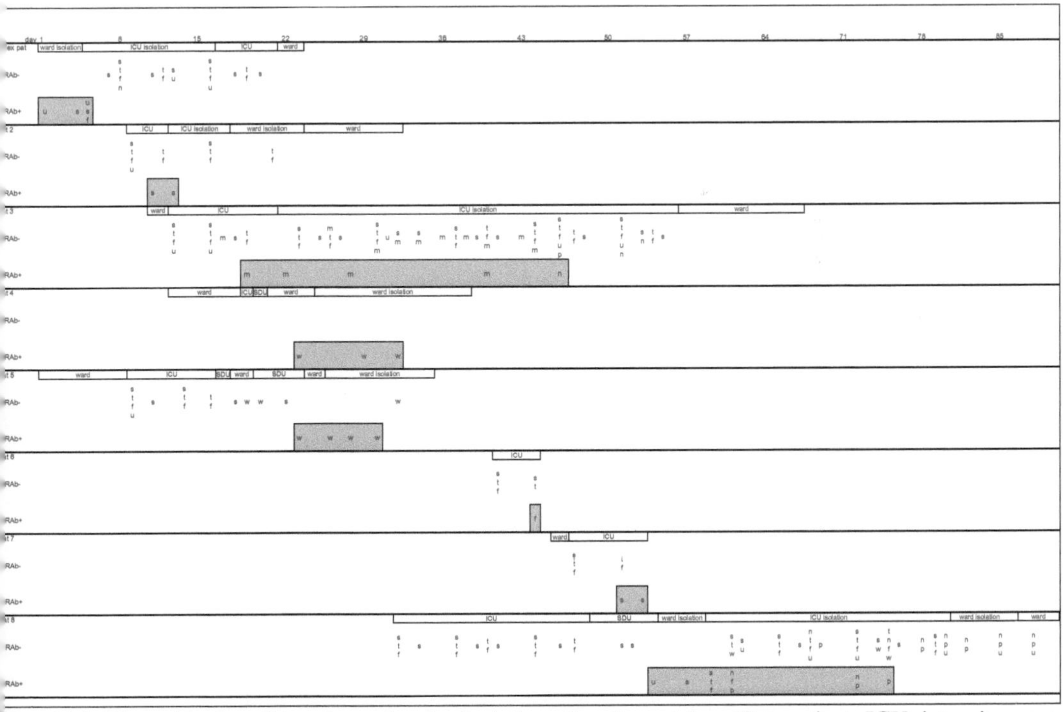

Fig. 11.1. Timetable describing the outbreak, depicting all cultures taken (Pat, patient; ICU, intensive care unit; SDU, step-down unit; MRAb-, no MRAb cultured from specified location or specimen; MRAB+, MRAb cultured from specified location or specimen; f, faeces or rectum; m, mediastinum; n, nose; p, perineum; s, sputum; t, throat; u, urine; w, wound)

Table 11.1 Comparison of patients who acquired multi-drug resistant *A. baumannii* with patients who were in the ICU during the outbreak but did not acquire MRAb. For patient 8 (see Table 11.2) only his first admission is taken in account, this being the period at risk for acquisition of MRAb (APACHE II, applied physiology and chronic health evaluation; Ventilated, intubated and artificially ventilated at any time during ICU stay; LOS, length of stay; NS, not significant; CI, confidence interval for the difference)

	Cases	Noninfected patients	*p*
No.	7	336	
Surgical/medical (*n*)	5/2	252/84	NS
Scheduled admission (*n*)	4	130	NS
Mean age (years)	62.8	63.1	NS
APACHE II (mean)	16.7	15.6	NS
LOS (mean, days)	12.7	2.5	<0.05
Ventilated (%)	100	97	<0.05
Hospital mortality (%)	28.6	13.7	NS

nasogastric or urethral catheters were removed or defaecation was induced [35] (Table 11.2). Environmental cultures yielded MRAb from several surfaces, including keyboards and telephones, but cultures from all healthcare workers involved were negative. The most remarkable feature of this outbreak was that only one patient acquired MRAb in the digestive tract—in this case MRAb was probably introduced by means of a rectal temperature probe. A second remarkable feature is the relatively small number of infected patients relative to earlier outbreaks with MRAb (Table 11.3) [1, 2, 27, 36-46]. SDD prevented digestive tract colonisation and subsequent secondary endogenous infection, but of course it did not prevent exogenous infection. It was already known that MRAb can survive for prolonged periods of time on dry surfaces with subsequent transfer to patients, but from our experience it can be learned that (1) digestive tract colonisation with subsequent infection can be prevented almost completely, (2) for eradication of MRAb from the digestive tract it may be necessary to induce defaecation in order for the nonresorbed antibiotics to reach the whole length of the gut, (3) MRAb can persist on nasogastric and probably also on oropharyngeal tubes, which must be replaced, (4) hand hygiene is still indispensable and (5) surveillance cultures pick up MRAb at an early stage and give insight into hygiene breaches.

ESBL and Tobramycin-Resistant Microorganisms

Extended-spectrum beta-lactamase (ESBL) producing AGNB have been reported several times in intensive care units that do not use SDD [36]. This phenomenon is related to the use of parenteral antimicrobials that suppress patient's indigenous flora of the digestive tract, thus promoting the subsequent over-

Table 11.2 Characteristics of patients secondarily colonised or infected with multi-drug resistant *Acinetobacter baumannii* (PTCA, percutaneous transluminal coronary angioplasty; IABP, intra-aortic balloon pump; AVR+MVR, aortic+mitral valve replacement; LVAD, left ventricular assist device; CABG, coronary artery bypass graft; LCO, low cardiac output; ICU/SDU- .., intensive care unit or step-down unit –[bed number]; imi-cil, imipenem-cilastin; ami, amikacin; PMX-neb, nebulisation of the lungs through endotracheal tube with polymyxin B; NA, not applicable)

Patient	2	3	4	5	6	7	8
Age (years)	54	55	76	64	42	80	73
Diagnosis	Myocardial infarction, urgent PTCA, IABP	AVR+MVR, IABP, LVAD, open mediastinum	CABG	CABG	Asphyxia	CABG, LCO	Myocardial infarction, urgent CABG, LCO
Unit and bed at probable time of colonisation	ICU-4	ICU-7	ICU-15 or SDU-22	SDU-22	ICU-11	ICU-9	ICU-10 or SDU-22
APACHE II score	23	9	14	13	20	16	22
Days in ICU before first MRAb isolation	2	7	1	9	3	5	17
Date of first MRAb isolation	Oct 20	Oct 28	Nov 1	Nov 1	Nov 22	Nov 29	Dec 2
Primary colonised site	Lungs	Mediastinum	Venectomy wound	Venectomy wound	Rectum	Lungs	Urine
Secondary colonised sites	-	Nose	-	-	-	Throat	Lungs, throat, nose, rectum, perineum
Infection / colonisation	Infection: pneumonia	Infection: mediastinitis	Colonisation	Colonisation	Colonisation	Infection: pneumonia	Infection: pneumonia
Specific treatment	imi-cil / ami / PMX-neb	imi-cil / ami / taurolidine irrigation	None	None	None	NA	imi-cil / ami / PMX-neb
Date of last MRAb-positive culture	Oct 22	Nov 24	Nov 7	Nov 8	NA	NA	Dec 23
Outcome	Survived	Survived	Survived	Survived	Died	Died	Survived
Comment	Admitted to original room of index patient, 6 days later	MRAb eliminated only after change of nasogastric tube	Stayed in ICU 1 day after CABG and 1 day in SDU; change of wound dressing in ICU; first wound culture 5 days after discharge from ICU	Stayed in ICU 9 days and in SDU 2 days after complicated CABG; readmitted to SDU for cardiac failure. Sputum, faeces and wound cultures negative at readmission to SDU, but later wound grew MRAb	Admitted after resuscitation for asphyxia; cultures at admission negative for MRAb; died of postanoxic encephalopathy. Culture taken on day of death positive for MRAb	Cultures at admission to ICU negative for MRAb; died of MRAb pneumonia before results of cultures were known	Discharged after 17 days ICU; cultures negative, no urine cultured; SDD discontinued; after 7 days SDU discharged to ward: MRAb in urine, isolation instituted. Readmitted to ICU with pneumonia. MRAb eliminated after change of the nasogastric tube and induced defaecation

Table 11.3 Comparison of reported ICU outbreaks of multi-drug resistant *Acinetobacter baumannii* (attrib mort, attributable mortality for MRAb acquisition; excess LOS, excess length of ICU stay in days for MRAb acquisition in ICU patients)

First author [ref.]	Colonised or infected patients (%)	Attrib mort (%)	Excess LOS
García-Garmendia [1]	4.6	30	13
Theaker [2]	7.8	11	3
Webster [36]	18.3	11	
Timsit [37]	14.1		
Scerpella [38]	14.3	25	13.5
Lortholary [39]	10.4	25	16
Crowe [40]	10		
Garrouste-Orgeas [41]	9.3		
Ayats [42]	66		
Corbella [27]	41	11	
D'Agata [43]	16		5
Koeleman [44]	10		
Aygün [45]	7		
Playford [46]	4.4	20	15
This study	2	15	10

growth of ESBL-producing AGNB in the gut [47, 48]. The combination of tobramycin and polymyxin E (colistin) orally and by gastric tube will prevent the persistence of ESBL producing AGNB. In addition, enteral tobramycin and polymyxin E (PT) will prevent overgrowth of AGNB. As overgrowth is the most important factor in the development of resistance, this can be prevented by enteral PT. In addition, outbreaks will more easily occur in the case of overgrowth than in the presence of low-level growth. In conclusion, enteral tobramycin and polymyxin E prevent overgrowth and thereby also outbreaks and the emergence of resistant microorganisms.

Al Naiemi et al. reported an outbreak of ESBL producing *E. coli* in patients treated with SDD [49]. However, there is no clear evidence in their report of transmission amongst the patients. The possibility of clonal mutation cannot be ruled out. The main problem in their report is not the emergence of the ESBL plasmid but the presence of tobramycin-resistant microorganisms. Polymyxin E alone has not been shown to clear AGNB successfully, irrespective of their resistance pattern [50]. All ESBL producing AGNB isolated within the first week of admission were resistant to tobramycin. This suggests they were present in the patient prior to admission, despite not being detected in the admission surveillance. In the case of tobramycin-resistant AGNB, adjustment of the PTA paste and suspension should be seriously considered. Neomycin [51] can be used, or otherwise paramomycin. The latter was used to control a multi-resistant *Serratia* endemicity in Spain (M.A. de la Cal, personal communication).

Methicillin-Resistant Staphylococcus aureus

SDD is not active against methicillin-resistant staphylococci. Parenteral vancomycin has never been shown to eradicate oropharyngeal and gastrointestinal MRSA carriage. Three recent trials have shown that enteral vancomycin is an effective and safe method of abolishing MRSA carriage and subsequent transmission and achieving control of an outbreak [11, 52, 53]. Topical therapy with vancomycin appears to be effective in preventing pneumonia, does not lead to vancomycin-resistant strains and is cost effective [54]. In addition to 500 mg q.i.d. of vancomycin enterally, a 4% gel in the oropharynx is used, as this appears to be more effective than a 2% gel [55]. Thus, the approach in the case of a patient with MRSA carrier status is to add vancomycin to the oral paste and suspension to eliminate the gastrointestinal reservoir. In addition, the nasal carriage is treated with locally applied mupirocin and the patient is washed twice daily with chlorhexidine to treat skin carriage. However, application of this policy does not result in complete elimination of MRSA: low concentrations are still present in the faeces. However, this concentration is low enough to prevent transmission after proper hand-washing.

The above studies screened rigorously for MRSA with intermediate sensitivity to vancomycin and for vancomycin-resistant enterococci [52, 53]. All samples, both diagnostic and surveillance, were negative for these two target microorganisms. Although vancomycin-resistant enterococci were imported into the Spanish ICU, extensive spread did not occur and no change in policy was required [52]. Finally, both trials show substantial savings to be offset in terms of the consumption of parenteral vancomycin, which was significantly reduced in both.

Yeast

Even the newer antifungals do not eradicate yeast overgrowth in the critically ill. In contrast, one RCT and one observational cohort study conducted in neonatal units demonstrated that enteral polyenes (amphotericin B and nystatin) control yeast outbreaks following the eradication of yeast overgrowth in critically ill patients [56, 57]. This is in line with the recent meta-analysis of RCTs on SDD, which has shown that the enteral component of amphotericin B significantly reduces fungal carriage and infection [58].

Conclusion

Outbreak control is based on the control of overgrowth. This is illustrated by the observation that AGNB can be completely eradicated from throat and gut, whilst low concentrations of MRSA and yeasts can still be detected in surveillance cultures after long-term administration of enteral vancomycin and polyenes.

Complete elimination will not be accomplished, but is also not necessary: the critical issue is prevention of overgrowth rather than complete elimination, as overgrowth causes secondary endogenous infection, transmission and the presence of resistant mutant. Surveillance cultures are indispensable in monitoring efficacy of SDD, emergence of abnormal flora including multi-resistant strains and control of hygiene.

Guidelines on Outbreak Control

Surveillance cultures of throat and rectum are indispensable in the management of an outbreak. Surveillance cultures are taken on admission and twice weekly thereafter (e.g. on Mondays and Thursdays). This type of samples allows detection of the carrier state of an outbreak strain, identification of the type of outbreak (endogenous vs exogenous) and monitoring of the efficacy of the manoeuvres implemented for outbreak control. Even in a unit in which SDD is not applied, routine cultures have proven to be very valuable in early detection of emerging resistance [12]. The outbreak studies discussed above all show that a delay in the administration of enteral antibiotics prolongs the outbreak [9, 52, 56]. All three studies show that immediate administration of enteral PTA and vancomycin to all patients requiring at least three days of ventilation effectively discontinues the outbreak.

Table 11.4 shows the doses of enteral microbial agents used in outbreak control.

Table 11.4 Doses of enterally administered antimicrobials used in outbreak control (dd: daily doses)l

First author [ref.]	Topical paste	Nasogastric tube	Intravenous antibiotics
Aerobic Gram-negative bacilli			
Taylor [10]	2% tobramycin, colistin, amphotericin B 6 dd oral/gum margins/nose/ rectum/vagina	Tobramycin 80 mg 6 dd; colistin Mu 6 dd Amphotericin B 500 mg 6 dd	
Brun-Buisson [9]		Nalidixic acid 1 g 4 dd Neomycin 1 g 4 dd Polymyxin E 50 mg 4 dd	
Methicillin-resistant *Staphylococcus aureus*			
De la Cal [52]	4% vancomycin 6 dd oral/tracheostomy/ pressure sores	Vancomycin 0.5 g 6 dd	
Silvestri [53]		Vancomycin 4 dd 0.5 g	
Thorburn [11]	2% vancomycin 4 dd oral	40 mg/kg/day	Cephradine
Yeasts			
Damnjanovic [56]	Nystatin solution by cotton swab oral	100,000 IU Nystatin	

If a multi-resistant strain has been present on admission it is advisable to remove and renew all foreign objects, such as nasogastric tubes, after administration of the suspension. This is especially important in the case of organisms that stick to surfaces, such as *Acinetobacter*. In patients affected by constipation, defaecation should be induced to allow the nonabsorbable antibiotics to cover the whole length of the digestive tract.

References

1. Garcia-Garmendia JL, Ortiz-Leyba C, Garnacho-Montero J, Jimenez-Jimenez FJ, Monterrubio-Villar J, Gili-Miner M (1999) Mortality and the increase in length of stay attributable to the acquisition of Acinetobacter in critically ill patients. Crit Care Med 27:1794-1799.
2. Theaker C, Azadian B, Soni N (2003) The impact of Acinetobacter baumannii in the intensive care unit. Anaesthesia 58:271-274.
3. CDC. Guidelines for Preventing Health-Care-Associated Pneumonia. http://www.cdc.gov/mmwr/preview/mmwrhtml/rr5303a1.htm accessed on 25 Feb. 2007
4. CDC. Guideline for Hand Hygiene in Health-Care Settings. Recommendations of the Health-care Infection Control Practices Advisory Committee and the HICPAC/SHEA/APIC/IDSA Hand Hygiene Task Force. http://www.cdc.gov/mmwr/preview/mmwrhtml/rr5116a1.htm Accessed on 25 Feb. 2007
5. Humphreys H, Towner KJ (1997) Impact of Acinetobacter spp. in intensive care units in Great Britain and Ireland. J Hosp Infect 37:281-286
6. Rashid A, Solomon LK, Lewis HG, Khan K (2006) Outbreak of epidemic methicillin-resistant Staphylococcus aureus in a regional burns unit: management and implications. Burns 32:452-457
7. Damjanovic V, Corbell X, van der Spoel JI, van Saene HKF (2005) Outbreaks of infection in intensive care units; usefulness of molecular techniques for outbreak analysis. In: van Saene H, Silvestri L, de la Cal M (eds) Infection control in intensive care units. Springer-Verlag Italia, Milan, pp 247-296
8. Damjanovic V, van Saene HK (2006) Polyclonal outbreaks: a story not yet told. J Hosp Infect 64:408-409
9. Brun-Buisson C, Legrand P, Rauss A, Richard C, Montravers F, Besbes M et al (1989) Intestinal decontamination for control of nosocomial multiresistant gram-negative bacilli. Study of an outbreak in an intensive care unit. Ann Intern Med 110:873-881
10. Taylor ME, Oppenheim BA (1991) Selective decontamination of the gastrointestinal tract as an infection control measure. J Hosp Infect 17:271-278
11. Thorburn K, Taylor N, Saladi SM, van Saene HK (2006) Use of surveillance cultures and enteral vancomycin to control methicillin-resistant Staphylococcus aureus in a paediatric intensive care unit. Clin Microbiol Infect 12:35-42
12. Johnson DR, Love-Dixon MA, Brown WJ, Levine DP, Downes FP, Hall WN (1992) Delayed detection of an increase in resistant Acinetobacter at a Detroit hospital. Infect Control Hosp Epidemiol 13:394-398
13. Husni RN, Goldstein LS, Arroliga AC, Hall GS, Fatica C, Stoller JK et al (1999) Risk factors for an outbreak of multi-drug-resistant Acinetobacter nosocomial pneumonia among intubated patients. Chest 115:1378-1382
14. Herruzo R, de la CJ, Fernandez-Acenero MJ, Garcia-Caballero J (2004) Two consecutive outbreaks of Acinetobacter baumannii 1-a in a burn intensive care unit for adults. Burns 30:419-423

15. Yu WL, Cheng HS, Lin HC, Peng CT, Tsai CH (2000) Outbreak investigation of nosocomial Enterobacter cloacae bacteraemia in a neonatal intensive care unit. Scand J Infect Dis 32:293-298
16. Cardoso CL, Pereira HH, Zequim JC, Guilhermetti M (1999) Effectiveness of hand-cleansing agents for removing Acinetobacter baumannii strain from contaminated hands. Am J Infect Control 27:327-331
17. Silvestri L, Petros AJ, Sarginson RE, de la Cal MA, Murray AE, van Saene HK (2005) Handwashing in the intensive care unit: a big measure with modest effects. J Hosp Infect 59:172-179
18. Schaberg DR, Weinstein RA, Stamm WE (1976) Epidemics of nosocomial urinary tract infection caused by multiply resistant gram-negative bacilli: epidemiology and control. J Infect Dis 133:363-366
19. Mulin B, Talon D, Viel JF, Vincent C, Leprat R, Thouverez M et al (1995) Risk factors for nosocomial colonization with multiresistant Acinetobacter baumannii. Eur J Clin Microbiol Infect Dis 14:569-576
20. Bonten MJ, Slaughter S, Ambergen AW, Hayden MK, van Voorhis J, Nathan C et al (1998) The role of "colonization pressure" in the spread of vancomycin-resistant enterococci: an important infection control variable. Arch Intern Med 158:1127-1132
21. Baines PB, Meyer J, de la Fuente JL (2001) Antimicrobial resistance in the intensive care unit: the use of oral non-absorbable antimicrobials may prolong the antibiotic are. Curr Anaesth Crit Care 12:41-47
22. Weist K, Pollege K, Schulz I, Ruden H, Gastmeier P (2002) How many nosocomial infections are associated with cross-transmission? A prospective cohort study in a surgical intensive care unit. Infect Control Hosp Epidemiol 23:127-132
23. Sanchez-Garcia M, Cambronero Galache JA, Lopez DJ, Cerda CE, Rubio BJ, Gomez Aguinaga MA et al (1998) Effectiveness and cost of selective decontamination of the digestive tract in critically ill intubated patients. A randomized, double-blind, placebo-controlled, multicenter trial. Am J Respir Crit Care Med 158:908-916
24. Villers D, Espaze E, Coste-Burel M, Giauffret F, Ninin E, Nicolas F et al (1998) Nosocomial Acinetobacter baumannii infections: microbiological and clinical epidemiology. Ann Intern Med 129:182-189
25. Lucet JC, Chevret S, Decre D, Vanjak D, Macrez A, Bedos JP et al (1996) Outbreak of multiply resistant Enterobacteriaceae in an intensive care unit: epidemiology and risk factors for acquisition. Clin Infect Dis 22:430-436
26. Simms HH, d'Amico R (1997) Posttraumatic auto-oxidative polymorphonuclear neutrophil receptor injury predicts the development of nosocomial infection. Arch Surg 132:171-172
27. Corbella X, Pujol M, Ayats J, Sendra M, Ardanuy C, Dominguez MA et al. (1996) Relevance of digestive tract colonization in the epidemiology of nosocomial infections due to multiresistant Acinetobacter baumannii. Clin Infect Dis 23:329-334
28. Podnos YD, Cinat ME, Wilson SE, Cooke J, Gornick W, Thrupp LD (2001) Eradication of multi-drug resistant Acinetobacter from an intensive care unit. Surg Infect (Larchmt) 2:297-301
29. Villegas MV, Hartstein AI (2003) Acinetobacter outbreaks, 1977-2000. Infect Control Hosp Epidemiol 24:284-295
30. Roberts SA, Findlay R, Lang SD (2001) Investigation of an outbreak of multi-drug resistant Acinetobacter baumannii in an intensive care burns unit. J Hosp Infect 48:228-232
31. Simor AE, Lee M, Vearncombe M, Jones-Paul L, Barry C, Gomez M et al (2002) An outbreak due to multiresistant Acinetobacter baumannii in a burn unit: risk factors for acquisition and management. Infect Control Hosp Epidemiol 23:261-267
32. Agusti C, Pujol M, Argerich MJ, Ayats J, Badia M, Dominguez MA et al (2002) Short-term effect of the application of selective decontamination of the digestive tract on different body site reservoir ICU patients colonized by multi-resistant Acinetobacter baumannii. J Antimicrob Chemother 49:205-208
33. de Jonge E, Schultz MJ, Spanjaard L, Bossuyt PM, Vroom MB, Dankert J et al (2003)

Effects of selective decontamination of digestive tract on mortality and acquisition of resistant bacteria in intensive care: a randomised controlled trial. Lancet 362:1011-1016

34. Nouira S, Elatrous S, Boukef R, Boujdaria R, Boussarsar M, Besbes L et al (1998) Effectiveness of selective digestive tract decontamination to control an outbreak of nosocomial pneumonia caused by Pseudomonas aeruginosa in mechanically ventilated patients. Clin Intensive Care 9:180-184
35. van der Spoel JI, Oudemans-van Straaten HM, Stoutenbeek CP, Bosman RJ, Zandstra DF (2001) Neostigmine resolves critical illness-related colonic ileus in intensive care patients with multiple organ failure—a prospective, double-blind, placebo-controlled trial. Intensive Care Med 27:822-827
36. Webster CA, Crowe M, Humphreys H, Towner KJ (1998) Surveillance of an adult intensive care unit for long-term persistence of a multi-resistant strain of Acinetobacter baumannii. Eur J Clin Microbiol Infect Dis 17:171-176
37. Timsit JF, Garrait V, Misset B, Goldstein FW, Renaud B, Carlet J (1993) The digestive tract is a major site for Acinetobacter baumannii colonization in intensive care unit patients. J Infect Dis 168:1336-1337
38. Scerpella EG, Wanger AR, Armitige L, Anderlini P, Ericsson CD (1995) Nosocomial outbreak caused by a multiresistant clone of Acinetobacter baumannii: results of the case-control and molecular epidemiologic investigations. Infect Control Hosp Epidemiol 16:92-97
39. Lortholary O, Fagon JY, Hoi AB, Slama MA, Pierre J, Giral P et al (1995) Nosocomial acquisition of multiresistant Acinetobacter baumannii: risk factors and prognosis. Clin Infect Dis 20:790-796
40. Crowe M, Towner KJ, Humphreys H (1995) Clinical and epidemiological features of an outbreak of acinetobacter infection in an intensive therapy unit. J Med Microbiol 43:55-62
41. Garrouste-Orgeas M, Chevret S, Arlet G, Marie O, Rouveau M, Popoff N et al (1997) Oropharyngeal or gastric colonization and nosocomial pneumonia in adult intensive care unit patients. A prospective study based on genomic DNA analysis. Am J Respir Crit Care Med 156:1647-1655
42. Ayats J, Corbella X, Ardanuy C, Dominguez MA, Ricart A, Ariza J et al (1997) Epidemiological significance of cutaneous, pharyngeal, and digestive tract colonization by multiresistant Acinetobacter baumannii in ICU patients. J Hosp Infect 37:287-295
43. D'Agata EM, Thayer V, Schaffner W (2000) An outbreak of Acinetobacter baumannii: the importance of cross-transmission. Infect Control Hosp Epidemiol 21:588-591
44. Koeleman JG, Parlevliet GA, Dijkshoorn L, Savelkoul PH, Vandenbroucke-Grauls CM (1997) Nosocomial outbreak of multi-resistant Acinetobacter baumannii on a surgical ward: epidemiology and risk factors for acquisition. J Hosp Infect 37:113-123
45. Aygun G, Demirkiran O, Utku T, Mete B, Urkmez S, Yilmaz M et al (2002) Environmental contamination during a carbapenem-resistant Acinetobacter baumannii outbreak in an intensive care unit. J Hosp Infect 52:259-262
46. Playford EG, Craig JC, Iredell JR (2007) Carbapenem-resistant Acinetobacter baumannii in intensive care unit patients: risk factors for acquisition, infection and their consequences. J Hosp Infect 65:204-211
47. Decré D, Gachot B, Lucet JC et al (1998) Clinical and bacteriologic epidemiology of extended-spetrum beta-lactamase-producing strains of Klebsiella pneumoniae in a medical intensive care unit. Clin Infect Dis 27:834-844
48. Pultz NJ, Stiefel U, Donskey CJ (2005) Effects of daptomycin, linezolid and vancomycin on establishment of intestinal colonization with vancomycin-resistant enterococci and extended-spectrum-b-lactamases-producing Klebsiella pneumoniae in mice. Antimicrob Agents Chemother 49:3513-3516
49. Al Naiemi N, Heddema ER, Bart A et al (2006) Emergence of multidrug-resistant Gram-negative bacteria during selective decontamination of the digestive tract on an intensive care unit. J Antimicrob Chemother 58:853-856
50. Sanchez M, Pizer BP, Alcock SR (2005) Enteral antimicrobials. In: van Saene HKF, Silvestri L, de la Cal MA (eds) Infection control in the intensive care unit, 2nd edn.. Springer-Verlag

Italia, Milan, pp 171-187

51. Brun-Buisson C, Legrand P, Rauss A et al (1989) Intestinal decontamination for control of nosocomial multiresistant gram-negative bacilli. Study of an outbreak in an intensive care unit. Ann Intern Med 110:873-881
52. de la Cal MA, Cerda E, van Saene HK, Garcia-Hierro P, Negro E, Parra ML et al (2004) Effectiveness and safety of enteral vancomycin to control endemicity of methicillin-resistant Staphylococcus aureus in a medical/surgical intensive care unit. J Hosp Infect 56:175-183
53. Silvestri L, Milanese M, Oblach L, Fontana F, Gregori D, Guerra R et al (2002) Enteral vancomycin to control methicillin-resistant Staphylococcus aureus outbreak in mechanically ventilated patients. Am J Infect Control 30:391-399
54. Silvestri L, van Saene HK, Milanese M, Fontana F, Gregori D, Oblach L et al (2004) Prevention of MRSA pneumonia by oral vancomycin decontamination: a randomised trial. Eur Respir J 23:921-926
55. Viviani M, van Saene HK, Dezzoni R, Silvestri L, Di Lenarda R, Berlot G et al (2005) Control of imported and acquired methicillin-resistant Staphylococcus aureus (MRSA) in mechanically ventilated patients: a dose-response study of enteral vancomycin to reduce absolute carriage and infection. Anaesth Intensive Care 33:361-372
56. Damjanovic V, Connolly CM, van Saene HK, Cooke RW, Corkill JE, van Belkum A et al (1993) Selective decontamination with nystatin for control of a Candida outbreak in a neonatal intensive care unit. J Hosp Infect 24:245-259
57. Sim ME, Yoo Y, You H, Salminen C, Walther FJ (1988) Prophylactic oral nystatin and fungal infections in very-low-birthweight infants. Am J Perinatol 5:33-36
58. Silvestri L, van Saene HK, Milanese M, Gregori D (2005) Impact of selective decontamination of the digestive tract on fungal carriage and infection: systematic review of randomized controlled trials. Intensive Care Med 31:898-910

Chapter 12
Preoperative Prophylaxis with SDD in Surgical Patients

Heleen M. Oudemans-van Straaten

Introduction

Selective decontamination of the digestive tract (SDD) in surgical patients is an antibiotic strategy to prevent perioperative endotoxaemia and postoperative infections. It does so by eradicating the carriage of aerobic Gram-negative bacilli (AGNB) and fungi in the digestive tract, from oropharynx to rectum [1], while sparing the anaerobic flora. High concentrations of potential pathogenic aerobic Gram-negative bacilli (AGNB) and fungi in the digestive tract may lead to the permeation of bacterial compounds such as endotoxins from the intestinal lumen to the blood, especially if the gut barrier is diminished, which may occur during surgery. The subsequent permeation of endotoxin contributes to a systemic inflammatory response syndrome after the operation [2, 3]. Abnormal colonisation of the digestive tract may also lead to infections in other organ sites, especially if the patient's immune competence is impaired [1]. Abolition of the carrier state may thus prevent gut-derived endotoxaemia and infections. The present contribution focuses on the preoperative use of SDD and discusses reasons for failure.

Search Strategy

To summarise the clinical trials, a systematic MEDLINE search was performed for controlled trials using the terms and text words 'selective decontamination', 'surgery', 'pancreatitis', 'endotoxin' and 'endotoxaemia'/'endotoxemia' in different combinations. Studies in which SDD was applied preoperatively were selected. Pancreatitis was included, because a substantial proportion of these patients undergo surgery in the course of their disease. SDD in patients undergoing liver transplantation is discussed in Chapter 13.

P.H.J. van der Voort, H.K.F. van Saene (eds.) *Selective Digestive Tract Decontamination in Intensive Care Medicine.*

Permeation of Intestinal Endotoxin from the Gut

Several factors contribute to the permeation of endotoxin from the intestinal lumen to patients' blood. Among these are intraluminal bacterial overgrowth, loss of gut barrier function and decreased competence of the gut-associated lymphoid tissue (GALT) [4, 5]. During surgery, several of these factors come into play. SDD controls bacterial overgrowth, but indirectly also attacks the gut barrier and immune competence of the GALT.

Interaction between Resident Intestinal Flora and Gut Barrier Function

The resident intestinal flora consists of more than 400 species of bacteria; there are 1,000 times as many anaerobes as aerobes. They form a microbial ecosystem containing more cells than the human body itself. This ecosystem protects against overgrowth of pathogenic bacteria. 'Colonisation resistance' is the term introduced by Van der Waay [6] to describe the protective role of the anaerobic resident flora. By the fermentation of fibre, anaerobes produce short-chain fatty acids that stimulate the colonic epithelium and the GALT, and induce tolerance [7, 8]. Fatty acids also inhibit the growth of nonindigenous AGNB. The healthy host develops specific secretory IgA against his/her resident flora, but has no specific immunity against hospital-acquired AGNB. Therefore, the resident flora forms the first-line defence against pathologic colonisation. Selectivity of the SDD regimen implies that PTA does not impact on the indigenous anaerobic flora.

Intraluminal bacterial (over)growth with nonindigenous flora and yeasts is a symptom of disease. It can result from the use of antibiotics, delayed intestinal motility, poor or absent enteral nutrition, poorly regulated diabetes mellitus and/or loss of immune competence. Abnormal colonisation with nonindigenous AGNB and yeasts is seen in a substantial proportion of elderly patients, hospitalised patients, and patients with diseases of the intestinal tract, malnutrition or decreased immune competence. Specific immunity for this nonindigenous flora is absent. If, in addition to overgrowth with nonindigenous flora, gut barrier function and the body's immune competence are compromised, the patient is at risk for gut-derived endotoxaemia and infections.

Nonspecific Gut Barrier Function

Loss of nonspecific gut barrier function can result from intestinal ischaemia and reperfusion, inflammatory mediators and enteral starvation [4]. In addition, overgrowth of nonindigenous microbes can induce a *local* inflammatory response with loss of barrier function and impaired anastomotic healing [9].

During surgery, intestinal ischaemia may occur as result of hypovolaemia and/or poor cardiac function. During cardiac surgery, the inflammatory response initiated by contact of patient's blood with nonendothelial surfaces in the extracorporeal circuit, as well as by reperfusion of the ischaemic heart and lungs, may also contribute to the loss of gut barrier function. Loss of gut barrier function during cardiac surgery is associated with endotoxaemia, postoperative hypermetabolism and clinical signs of inflammation [2, 3]. Severe acute pancreatitis is also associated with an early increase in intestinal permeability and endotoxaemia [10].

An interaction between intraluminal bacteria and gut barrier function becomes obvious in several ways. In a rat model, following total gastrectomy, SDD provided protection against anastomotic insufficiency [9]. Anastomotic insufficiency was associated with the presence of bacteria and pus. The proposed mechanism is that the bacterial endo- or exotoxins cause macrophage-mediated down-regulation of fibroblast proliferation. Proliferation of bacteria in necrotic tissue in the suture line may lead to the formation of intramural abscess formation. Local infection and the associated release of bacterial toxins and inflammatory mediators may increase the necrosis associated with microcirculatory disturbance at the suture line and impair healing. In the setting of cardiac surgery, the degree of endotoxaemia during surgery was lower and the gastric intramucosal pH (pHi) declined less markedly in patients treated with SDD preoperatively than in control patients. Factors associated with endotoxaemia were the concentration of AGNB, gastric pHi, duration of cardiopulmonary bypass and type of flow. In multiple logistic regression analysis, the concentration of AGNB and the type of flow emerged as significant determinants of endotoxaemia [11].

Factors Contributing to the Success of SDD

For SDD to be successful in reducing both endotoxaemia and infections caused by Gram-negative bacilli and fungi, several requirements have to be fulfilled [1, 12]. First, it is crucial that the correct antibiotics are used. Secondly, the antibiotics have to be administered for a sufficient number of days, and the patient has to be free of AGNB and fungi. To attain adequate decontamination, measures may have to be taken to stimulate intestinal motility and defaecation. The drug should have a spectrum covering all Enterobacteriaceae while sparing the resident anaerobes; it should not be inactivated by low pH; and it should bind minimally to food and faeces. To reach high intraluminal concentrations, the drug should not be absorbed or have a high degree of biliary and mucosal excretion as is the case with quinolones. Absorption of oral antibiotics without subsequent enteral excretion may give subtherapeutic systemic concentrations, leading to selection of resistant strains [13]. Thirdly, the ideal drug should have anti-endotoxin effects [12]. Only the classic regimen using polymyxin, tobramycin and amphotericin (PTA) has been shown to reduce endotoxaemia. Finally, surveillance cultures have to be taken for staff to become aware of persistent colonisation attributable to inadequate application of the drugs or possible growth of resistant microorganisms.

Explanations for Failure of Preoperative SDD

Explanations for the failure of preoperative SDD can be derived from what has been said above. Inactivation of the antibiotics by faecal material varies widely with different regimens [13, 14]. Tobramycin, ciprofloxacin and ofloxacin are affected minimally, gentamicin and polymyxin moderately and neomycin heavily. In faeces, tobramycin is much more potent than polymyxin and neomycin, or polymyxin and gentamicin. The combination of polymyxin and tobramycin gives the best results [1].

The efficacy of the different SDD regimens in eradicating AGNB does not go hand in hand with their efficacy in neutralising endotoxins. Both animal and human studies have shown that there is no correlation between faecal endotoxin levels and AGNB concentrations [15]. Eradication of AGNB does not guarantee adequate neutralisation of endotoxins. During the initial phase of gut decontamination, faecal endotoxin levels rise, while the degree of the rise depends on the antibiotics used. In the first five hours after the administration of either polymyxin plus tobramycin or ciprofloxacin via a duodenal tube to immune-compromised rats challenged with live *E. coli*, maximum endotoxin levels in plasma of the rats treated with polymyxin plus tobramycin were double those in controls, and plasma endotoxin levels in the rats treated with ciprofloxacin were 5–6 times control levels [16]. During the first week of SDD with neomycin, suppression of the coliform count with streptomycin and amphotericin was even associated with a 30-fold rise in faecal endotoxin concentration [17]. This rise in faecal endotoxin after antibiotic exposure may be explained by the antibiotic-mediated release of endotoxin. The extent of the reduction in faecal endotoxin after achievement of an AGNB-free carrier status depends on the decontaminating agents used [18]. In contrast to polymyxin and tobramycin [18], neomycin failed to show any anti-endotoxin properties in faeces [17]. Although polymyxin is a potent endotoxin binder, polymyxin alone reduced faecal endotoxin by a factor of 10, whilst the combination of polymyxin and tobramycin reduced intestinal endotoxin concentrations by 10^4 [18]. Since polymyxin is inactivated by faeces to a higher extent than tobramycin [1], its use may result in faecal levels that are sufficiently lethal against live AGNB but too low to further neutralise 'free' endotoxin. It is therefore necessary to add tobramycin to polymyxin to obtain a significant reduction in faecal endotoxin. The mechanism of the low endotoxin release accompanying bacterial killing by tobramycin has not been fully explained. It may be related to the lack of cell wall destruction rather than to endotoxin binding [19]. In contrast to tobramycin, the addition of ciprofloxacin to bacterial cultures in vitro caused significant endotoxin release

[19,20]. The use of ciprofloxacin for SDD, although adequate for bacterial killing, is likely to be associated with an initial increase in gut endotoxin.

Results of Prospective Randomised Trials

Several randomised trials have been conducted in humans to evaluate the effect of preoperative SDD. Three main groups of patients were studied: patients undergoing cardiac surgery [11, 21], patients undergoing oesophageal, gastric or colon resection [22–24], and patients with severe pancreatitis [25]. The end-points of these studies varied in the different populations. In the cardiac surgery patients, endotoxaemia and inflammatory response were the main end-points. In those undergoing upper and lower intestinal surgery, reduction of postoperative infections was the primary target, while anastomotic leakage [24] and length of stay in the ICU [23] were also studied. In patients with severe pancreatitis, post-operative infections and clinical outcomes were the end-points of study. Results of prospective randomised human trials on endotoxaemia are summarised in Table 12.1, and those of the randomised trials on postoperative infections and clinical outcomes, in Table 12.2.

Table 12.1 Randomised controlled trials (RCT) of preoperative SDD on endotoxaemia (PTA, polymyxin E 100 mg, tobramycin 80 mg, amphotericin 500 mg; PN, polymyxin B 500,000 U [50 mg], neomycin 125 mg)

First author [ref.] year	Study design	No. of patients SDD control	Population	SDD regimen	Duration of SDD before surgery (days)	Perioperative endotoxaemia cytokinaemia
Martinez Pellus [11] 1997	RCT, unblinded	50–50	Cardiac surgery	PTA q.i.d.	3	Significant decrease
Bouter [21] 2002	RCT, blinded	51–27	Cardiac surgery	PN q.i.d.	5-7	No decrease

Effect on Endotoxaemia

Of the two randomised trials evaluating the effect of preoperative SDD on endotoxaemia and associated cytokine release during cardiac surgery, one was positive [11]. In this trial, the classic PTA regimen [26] was used in an adequate dose and for a sufficient number of days. There are several explanations for the failure of SDD to reduce endotoxaemia in the other trial [21]. In this study, the dose of polymyxin used was half the known effective dose, neomycin was used instead of tobramycin and no antifungal therapy was applied. In contrast with tobramycin, neomycin fails to show any anti-endotoxin properties in faeces [17].

Table 12.2 RCT of preoperative SDD and its influence on infections, anastomotic leakage and mortality (PTA, polymyxin E 100 mg, tobramycin 80 mg, amphotericin 500 mg; PTVA, polymyxin B 100 mg, tobramycin 80 mg, vancomycin 125 mg, amphotericin 500 mg; CNA, colistin sulphate 200 mg, norfloxacin 50 mg and amphotericin 500 mg)

First author [ref.] year	Study design	No. of patients–no. of SDD controls	Population	SDD regimen; preoperative duration	Systemic antibiotics, SDD control	Infections Other clinical outcomes
Tetteroo [22] 1990	RCT, unblinded	56–58	Oesophageal resection	PTA q.i.d.; 3 days	Cefotaxime + metronidazol, cefamandol + metronidazol	Fewer pulmonary and wound infections
Taylor [23] 1994	RCT, unblinded	189–192	Elective colorectal surgery	Ciprofloxacin 500 mg b.i.d. + purgative; 1 day	Piperacillin 4 g once	Fewer wound infections, abdominal abscesses and cases of sepsis
Shardey [24] 1997	RCT, blinded	102–103	Total gastrectomy	PTVA q.i.d.; 1 day	Cefotaxime twice	Fewer pulmonary infections and cases of anastomotic leakage
Luiten [25] 1995	RCT, unblinded	50–52	Severe pancreatitis	CNA q.i.d. + oral paste + rectal enema	SDD: cefotaxime[a] controls: Infection guided	Fewer pancreatic infections, fewer laparotomies, lower mortality in severe pancreatitis

[a]Until AGNB were eliminated from the oral cavity and rectum

Effect on Postoperative Infections, Anastomotic Leakage and Clinical Outcome

In all three randomised clinical trials conducted in patients undergoing upper and lower intestinal surgery, the use of preoperative SDD resulted in fewer post-operative infections. In the study published by Schardey, SDD also reduced the incidence of anastomotic leakage [24]. In this trial, vancomycin was added to the PTA regimen. In the Scottish multicentre trial, length of stay in the hospital was significantly shorter in the SDD-treated patients [23]. It should be noted that in this trial, SDD consisted of ciprofloxaxin 500 mg twice daily and was applied only preoperatively in combination with a purgative.

In a multicentre RCT, Luiten studied 102 patients with early severe pancreatitis [25]. The SDD regimen consisted of oral antibiotics that the patients had to swallow and local application in the oral cavity of a sticky paste containing 2% of the antibiotics, each four times daily, and administration of the same antibiotics in a rectal enema once daily (Table 12.2). It should be noted that the SDD patients received systemic cefotaxime in addition until AGNB were eliminated from the oral cavity and rectum, whereas the control patients received antibiotics only when concurrent infection was present. The pancreatic infection rate was significantly lower in the SDD patients. All cases with Gram-negative pancreatic infection had had preceding colonisation of the digestive tract with identical microorganisms. Fewer laparotomies were required in SDD patients than in controls. The difference in mortality between the groups (22% in the SDD group vs 35% in the controls) was only significant after correction for severity of pancreatitis.

Conclusion

It is concluded that preoperative SDD can be an effective tool in reducing endotoxaemia, always providing that it is applied with the proper antibiotics in sufficient doses and over an adequate period. Otherwise, an anti-endotoxin effect of SDD is unlikely. Only the combination of polymyxin 100 mg, tobramycin 80 mg and amphotericin 500 mg (PTA) applied four times daily for three days has been shown to reduce endotoxaemia in cardiac surgery patients.

The evidence that preoperative use of SDD reduces postoperative infections following oesophageal, gastric or colon resection is strong. The use of preoperative SDD is recommended in patients undergoing these surgical operations. In this population, SDD may also prevent anastomotic leakage and shorten the stay in hospital. The single RCT of SDD in acute severe pancreatitis shows that SDD reduces the frequency of secondary pancreatic infections and the need for laparotomy, and its results suggest that SDD may reduce mortality. It should be noted, however, that the SDD regimen applied in this trial included an initial short course of i.v. cefotaxime.

References

1. Stoutenbeek CP, Van Saene HKF (1990) Infection prevention in intensive care by selective decontamination of the digestive tract. J Crit Care 5:137-156
2. Oudemans-van Straaten HM, Jansen PGM, Te Velthuis H et al (1996) Increased oxygen consumption after cardiac surgery is associated with the inflammatory response to endotoxemia. Intensive Care Med 22:294-300
3. Oudemans-van Straaten HM, Jansen PGM, Hoek FJ et al (1996) Intestinal permeability, circulating endotoxin and post-operative systemic responses in cardiac surgery patients. J Thorac Cardiovasc Anesthesia 10:187-194
4. Unno N, Fink MP (1998) Intestinal epithelial hyperpermeability. Mechanism and relevance to disease. Gastroenteral Clin North Am 127:289-307
5. DeWitt RC, Kudsk KA (1999) The gut's role in metabolism, mucosal barrier function, and gut immunology. Infect Dis Clin North Am 13:465-481
6. Waay van der D, Berghuis-de Vries JM, Lekkerkerk van der Wees JEC (1972) Colonization resistance of the digestive tract of mice during systemic antibiotic treatment. J Hyg (Lond) 70:605-610
7. Chapman MAS (2001) The role of the colonic flora in maintaining a healthy large bowel mucosa. Ann R Coll Surg Engl 83:75-80
8. Hooper LV, Gordon JI (2001) Commensal host-bacterial relationships in the gut. Science 292:1115-1118
9. Schardey HM, Kamps T, Rau HG et al (1994) Bacteria: a major pathogenic factor for anastomotic insufficiency. Antimicrob Agents Chemother 38:2564-2567
10. Ammori BJ, Becker KL, Kite P et al (2003) Calcitonin precursors: early markers of gut barrier dysfunction in patients with acute pancreatitis. Pancreas 27:239-243
11. Martinez-Pellús AF, Merino P, Bru M et al (1997) Endogenous endotoxemia of intestinal origin during cardiopulmonary bypass. Role of the type of flow and the protective effect of selective digestive decontamination. Intensive Care Med 23:1251-1257
12. Oudemans-van Straaten HM, Van Saene HKF, Zandstra DF (2003) Selective decontamination of the digestive tract, use of the correct antibiotics is crucial. Crit Care Med 31:334-335
13. Van Saene JJM, Van Saene HKF, Stoutenbeek CP et al (1985) Influence of faeces on the activity of antimicrobial agents used for decontamination of the alimentary canal. Scand J Infect Dis 17:295-300
14. Van Saene HK, Lemmens SE, Van Saene JJ (1988) Gut decontamination by oral ofloxacin and ciprofloxacin in healthy volunteers. J Antimicrob Chemother 22 Suppl C:127-134
15. Van Saene JJM, Stoutenbeek CP, Van Saene HKF (1992) Faecal endotoxin in human volunteers: normal values. Microb Ecol Health Dis 5:179-184
16. Schulze C, Oesser S, Hein H et al (2001) Risk of endotoxemia during the initial phase of gut decontamination with antimicrobial agents. Res Exp Med (Berl) 200:169-174
17. Rogers MJ, Moore R, Cohen J (1985) The relationship between faecal endotoxin and faecal microflora of the C57BL mouse. J Hyg Contrib 95:397-402
18. Van Saene JJM, Stoutenbeek CP, Van Saene HKF et al (1996) Reduction of the intestinal endotoxin pool by three different SDD regimens in human volunteers. J Endotoxin Res 3:337-343
19. Crosby HA, Bion JF, Penn CW et al (1994) Antibiotic-induced release of endotoxin from bacteria in vitro. J Med Microbiol 40:23-30
20. Sjölin J, Goscinski G, Lundholm M et al (2000) Endotoxin release from Escherichia coli after exposure to tobramycin: dose-dependency and reduction in cefuroxime-induced endotoxin release. Clin Microbiol Infect 6:74-81
21. Bouter H, Schippers E, Luelmo SAC et al (2002) No effect of preoperative selective gut decontamination on endotoxemia and cytokine activation during cardiopulmonary bypass: a randomized, placebo-controlled study. Crit Care Med 30:38-43

22. Tetteroo GW, Wagenvoort JH, Ince C et al (1990) Effects of selective decontamination on gram-negative colonisation, infections and development of bacterial resistance in esophageal resection. Intensive Care Med 16 Suppl 3:S224-228
23. Taylor EW, Lindsay G (1994) Selective decontamination of the colon before elective colorectal surgery. West of Scotland Surgical Infection Study Group. World J Surg 18:926-931
24. Schardey HM, Joosten U, Finke U et al (1997) The prevention of anastomotic leakage after total gastrectomy with local decontamination. A prospective, randomized, double-blind, placebo-controlled multicenter trial. Ann Surg 225:172-180
25. Luiten EJ, Hop WC, Lange JF et al (1995) Controlled clinical trial of selective decontamination for the treatment of severe acute pancreatitis. Ann Surg 222:57-65
26. Stoutenbeek CP, van Saene HKF, Miranda DR et al (1984) The effect of selective decontamination of the digestive tract on colonisation and infection rate in multiple trauma patients. Intensive Care Med 10:1851-1892

Chapter 13
The Role of SDD in Liver Transplantation: a Meta-Analysis

Peter H.J. van der Voort and Hendrick K.F. van Saene

Introduction and rationale

Wiesner et al. introduced SDD as infection prophylaxis in liver transplantation in 1987 and 1988 [1, 2]. These investigators reasoned that liver transplant recipients are the prime subset of patients to benefit from SDD prophylaxis for three reasons:

1. Liver transplant recipients are at high risk of infection
2. Most infections are endogenous following gut overgrowth
3. The potential pathogens causing infection in liver transplant recipients are aerobic Gram-negative bacilli (AGNB) and yeasts, the target microorganisms of SDD.

Liver transplant recipients are well known to be immunoparalysed owing to their underlying liver disease. Their immunity is suppressed following surgery that involves intestinal manipulation and reduction of intestinal blood flow. They invariably receive immunosuppressive medication and require endotracheal intubation immediately after receiving their liver transplants. Often there is no enteral feeding, a well-known risk factor for overgrowth and subsequent endogenous infections [3].

Most infections in liver transplant recipients have an endogenous origin. These patients develop infections with the potential pathogens they carry in throat and gut in overgrowth concentrations. A distinction should be made between major and minor infections. Major infections are defined as infections with severe morbidity requiring antimicrobial therapy and include septicaemia, peritonitis, abscesses and pneumonia. In contrast, minor infections are characterised by minimal morbidity, such as asymptomatic bacteriuria, superficial wound infection, colonisation of bile and contamination of the T-tube [4].

In the first month after transplantation, recipients are at high risk of AGNB and yeast infections, whilst viral infections are predominant in the second and third months after transplantation [5]. Patients with chronic underlying conditions, including liver disease, carry abnormal flora such as AGNB and yeasts, and 35% of hospitalised patients with cirrhosis carry *Klebsiella, Enterobacter*

P.H.J. van der Voort, H.K.F. van Saene (eds.) *Selective Digestive Tract Decontamination in Intensive Care Medicine.* © Springer 2008

and *Citrobacter* species in the gut [6]. This preoperative abnormal flora causes early primary endogenous infections after transplantation. ICU- and hospital-acquired AGNB are responsible for secondary endogenous and exogenous infections after one week of transplantation.

These observations justify the assessment of SDD as surgical prophylaxis in liver transplant recipients and its use for one month after transplantation in view of the ongoing immunoparalysis [7].

Search strategy and selection criteria

We searched for published reports on PubMed, Medline and Embase. The keywords we used were 'SDD', 'liver disease', and 'liver transplantation'. No limits were set for search criteria, although we gave preference to randomised and other studies published in peer-reviewed journals. We did not exclude articles in other languages as long as there was an English abstract.

Results of literature search

A total of eighteen studies involving a total of 1,657 patients were retrieved from the literature published between 1987 and 2004 [4, 5, 8–23]. Nine studies were observational, six were randomised controlled trials (RCTs) and three had historical controls; seven trials were conducted in North American transplant units, three in The Netherlands, two trials each in Spain and Germany, and one study each in Italy, UK, Belgium and Denmark. Table 13.1 shows the data recorded in all eighteen studies. Table 13.2 shows the parenteral and enteral protocols used in the six RCTs. The enteral strategy invariably comprised of polymyxin, an antipseudomonal aminoglycoside and a polyene. The enteral antibiotics were applied in both oropharynx and gut, except in one German trial in which only enteral antibiotics were administered. Table 13.3 shows the sample size and the infection and mortality rates in both test and control groups. The six randomised trials include 363 liver transplant patients. However, the number of patients with infections who could be included in the meta-analysis was 317. There was a significant difference in infection rate (number of infected patients) in the study of Bion. A comparison of the total number of infections is reported in some studies, but the number of infected patients is preferred. Mortality data were reported in all but two trials. There was no difference in mortality between test and control groups in any of the trials. This is due to a low baseline mortality rate and to the limited number of patients included in each study (type II error).

Table 13.1 Data recorded in all eighteen studies yielded by the literature search (Observ: observational study; Histor: historical control group; Random: randomised controlled trial. AGNB: aerobic Gram-negative bacteria)

First author	Journal, year	Design	Patients		Infected patients No.		Infected patients Percentage	
			Control	Test	Control	Test	Control	Test
Cuervas-Mons [8]	Transplant Proc, 1989	Observ	—	23	—	9	—	39
Wiesner [4]	Infection, 1990	Observ	—	145	—	37	—	26
Van Zeijl [9]	Infection, 1990	Observ	—	10	—	6	—	60
Rosman [10]	Transplant Proc, 1990	Observ	—	39	—	19	—	42
Corti [11]	Transplant Proc, 1991	Observ	—	46	—	31	—	69
Gorensek [12]	Cleve Clin J Med, 1993	Histor	34	17	18	1	53 AGNB	6 AGNB
Smith [13]	Transplantation, 1993	Random	18	18	11	3	50 AGNB	11 AGNB
Bion [14]	Crit Care Med, 1994	Random	32	27	12	3	37.5	11
Steffen [15]	Transplant Int, 1994	Observ	—	191	—	57	—	28
Decruyenaere 16]	Transplant Proc, 1995	Observ	—	85	—	3	— Fungi	4 Fungi
Arnow [17]	Clin Infect Dis, 1996	Random	33	36	14, 12	14, 6	42, 36	39, 23
Kuo [18]	Am J Surgery, 1997	Histor	18	18	11	7	61.1	38.8
Hjortrup [19]	Transplant Proc, 1997	Observ	—	150	—	72	—	48
Emre [20]	Mt Sinai J Med, 1997	Histor	157	212	69	56	44	26
Hellinger [21]	Transplantation, 2002	Random	43	37	12	12	27.9	32.4
Zwaveling [22]	Crit Care Med, 2002	Random	29	26	25	22	86	84.5
Rayes [23]	Transplantation, 2002	Random	32	32	11	15	34	48
Losada [5]	Enferm Infecc, 2002	Observ	—	149	11	109	—	73.1

Table 13.2 SDD regimens in liver transplant RCTs (A, amphotericin B; AGNB, aerobic Gram-negative bacteria; ampicillin; I, intestinal; metro, metronidazole; Ny, nystatin; PT, O, oropharyngeal; PG, polymyxin E and gentamicin; PT, polymyxin E and tobramycin)

First author [ref.]	Parenteral	Enteral			
		AGNB	Yeasts	*S. aureus*	Site
Smith [13]	Cefotax/ampi, 2 arms	PT	A	—	O, I
Bion [12]	Cefotax/ampi, 2 arms	PT	A 2 arms	—	O, I
Arnow [15]	Cefotax/ampi, 2 arms	PG	Ny	—	O, I
Hellinger [21]	Ceftizoxime, 2 arms	PG	Ny 2 arms	—	O, I
Rayes [23]	Ceftriaxon/metro, 2 arms	PT	A	—	-, I
Zwaveling [22]	Cefotax/tobra, 2 arms	PT	A	—	O, I

Table 13.3 Infection and mortality data in six RCTs in liver transplantation patients

First author [ref.]	Sample size		Infection rate		Mortality rate	
	Test	Control	Test	Control	Test	Control
Smith [13]	18	18	3	11	2	3
Bion [12]	27	32	3	12	0	5
Arnow [15]	26	33	11	14	3	3
Hellinger [21]	37	43	12	12	2	2
Rayes [23]	32	32	15	11	Not mentioned	
Zwaveling [22]	26	29	22	25	Not mentioned	
Total	148	169				

Meta-Analyses

Two meta-analyses are available in the literature [24, 25]. The first is a Canadian one analysing three RCTs. The second, North American, meta-analysis evaluates four RCTs. The overall infection rate in the first meta-analysis was significantly lower in the liver transplant recipients who received SDD, with an odds ratio of 0.44 (95% CI 0.25-0.87). The second meta-analysis found a significantly reduced relative risk of 0.16 (95% 0.07-0.37) for patients with infections attributable to the target microorganisms AGNB and yeasts [25]. However, the difference in relative risk was no longer significant when all infections were analysed. The differences in number of infected patients and of episodes of infection were no longer significant owing to a higher number of episodes of infection with the low-level pathogens enterococci and coagulase-negative staphylococci. No distinction was made between major infections, such as pneumonia and septicaemia, and minor infections, including superficial wound infection and even bile colonisation diluting the net impact of SDD. In addition, the definitions applied for wound and bile infections relied on vague terms such as 'positive culture' and 'infected bile'. Patients do not usually die of enterococcal and coagulase-negative staphylococcal contamination of the T-tube, but they do generally succumb to pseudomonal and fungal sepsis. These invasive infections were completely prevented by SDD in both meta-analyses.

We performed a meta-analysis of all six RCTs. Figure 13.1 shows the analysis of the number of patients with any infection, whether of Gram-negative, Gram-positive or yeast origin. Excluded from this analysis is the study by Smith, as the total number of infections is not reported for this one. Figure 13.1 shows that the total number of infections was not reduced.

Figure 13.2 shows the analysis of the numbers of patients with AGNB or yeast infection. The studies by Zwaveling and Bion are excluded from this analysis, as the reports do not give these data, though they do report the total number of AGNB or yeast infections. However, Zwaveling et al. report that in their study the total number of infections caused by AGNB or yeasts was significantly lower in the SDD-treated group of patients.

Figures 13.1 and 13.2 show that SDD does reduce the frequency of infections by PPM such as AGNB and yeasts, as it is designed to. Apparently, more infections with low-level pathogens are reported, but the definitions for wound and bile infections relying on such vague terms as positive culture and infected bile are unsatisfactory [22]. Moreover, Zwaveling et al. do not specify the Gram-positive microorganisms as the potential pathogen *Staphylococcus aureus* or the

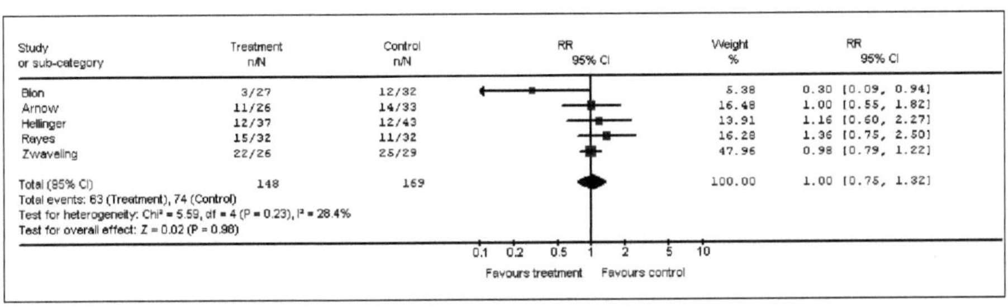

Fig. 13.1 Meta-analysis of all infections in liver transplant patients treated with or without SDD

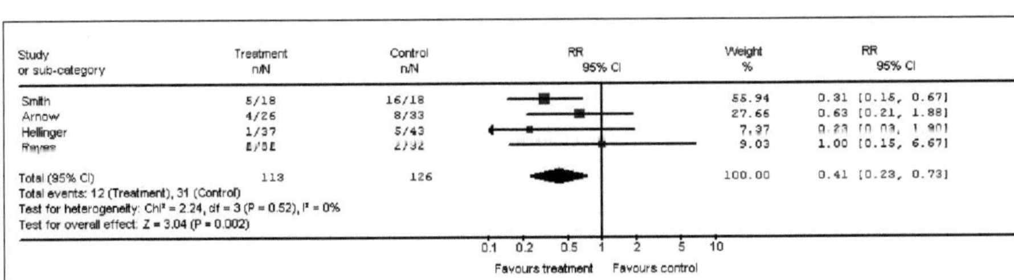

Fig. 13.2 Meta-analysis of AGNB and yeast infections in liver transplant patients treated with or without SDD

low-level pathogens enterococci and coagulase-negative staphylococci. Patients do not usually die of enterococcal and coagulase-negative staphylococcal wound infections, but they do generally succumb because of pseudomonal and fungal sepsis.

In conclusion, the number of patients with AGNB or yeast infection is significantly decreased by SDD. Prevention of these infections is the target of SDD. It cannot be expected to reduce the frequency of infections with Gram-positive bacteria, in particular enterococci and coagulase-negative staphylococci. On the other hand, *S. aureus* infections are prevented, as both cefotaxime and PTA are effective against *S. aureus* (see Chapter 2).

Antimicrobial Resistance

All reports of RCTs in patients undergoing liver transplantation that provide information on resistance explicitly state that there were no infections attributable to resistant AGNB. This finding is in line with the findings of the most recent meta-analysis of SDD, dealing with thirty-six RCTs conducted over seventeen years, which showed that antibiotic resistance was not a clinical problem. The latest RCT, evaluating SDD in about 1,000 patients requiring treatment in ICUs, found significantly fewer carriers of multiresistant AGNB in patients receiving SDD than in the control group [26]. In contrast, a recent observational study using quinolones, in particular norfloxacin, instead of polymyxin/tobramycin, in 149 liver transplant patients revealed a substantial infection rate due to norfloxacin-resistant AGNB and MRSA [5]. The proportion of AGNB, in particular *Pseudomonas aeruginosa*, resistant to norfloxacin was 38.8%. The mechanism of preventing resistance relies on the fact that high levels of the nonabsorbable antibiotics polymyxin/tobramycin in saliva and faeces in combination with the synergistic antibiotic effect and the maintenance of colonisation resistance create a unique environment that has proved strikingly successful in preventing overgrowth of resistant mutants among the target microorganisms.

Conclusion

In conclusion, preoperative prophylaxis with enteral polymyxin, tobramycin and amphotericin B combined with a short course of parenteral cefotaxime has been shown to be effective in reducing Gram-negative and yeast infections in liver transplant patients. In addition, it has been shown to be a safe protocol as far as antimicrobial resistance is concerned in patients receiving a liver transplant. If the liver transplant candidate starts on SDD when a liver becomes available this is soon enough.

References

1. Wiesner RH, Hermans P, Rakela J et al (1987) Selective bowel decontamination to prevent gram-negative bacterial and fungal infection following orthotopic liver transplantation. Transplant Proc 19(1 Pt 3):2420-2423
2. Wiesner RH, Hermans PE, Rakela J et al (1988) Selective bowel decontamination to decrease gram-negative aerobic bacterial and Candida colonization and prevent infection after orthotopic liver transplantation. Transplantation 45:570-574
3. Arnow PM (1995) Prevention of bacterial infection in the transplant recipient. The role of selective bowel decontamination. Infect Dis Clin North Am 9:849-862
4. Wiesner RH (1990) The incidence of Gram-negative bacterial and fungal infections in liver transplant patient treated with selective decontamination. Infection 18 [Suppl 1]:S19-S21
5. Losada I, Cuervas-Mons V, Damaso IMD (2002) Infeccion precoz en el paciente con trasplante hepatico: incidencia, gravedad, factores de riesgo y sensibilidad antibiotica de los aislados bacterianos. Enferm Infecc Microbiol Clin 20:422-430
6. Dupeyron C, Mangeney N, Sedrati L et al (1994) Rapid emergence of quinolone resistance in cirrhotic patients treated with norfloxacin to prevent spontaneous bacterial peritonitis. Antimicrob Agents Chemother 38:340-344
7. van Saene HKF, Zandstra DF (2004) Selective decontamination of the digestive tract: rationale behind evidence based use in liver transplantation. Liver Transpl 10:828-833
8. Cuervas-Mons V, Barrios C, Garrido A et al (1989) Bacterial infections in liver transplant patients under selective decontamination with norfloxacin. Transplant Proc 21:3558
9. van Zeijl JH, Kroes ACM, Metselaar HJ et al (1990) Infections after auxiliary partial liver transplantation. Experiences in the first ten patients. Infection 18:146-151
10. Rosman C, Klompmaker IJ, Bonsel GJ et al (1990) The efficacy of selective bowel decontamination as infection prevention after liver transplantation. Transplant Proc 22:1554-1555
11. Corti A, Sabbadini D, Pannacciulli, E et al (1991) Early severe infections after othotopic liver transplantation. Transplant Proc 23:1964
12. Gorensek MJ, Carey WD, Washington JA et al (1993) Selective bowel decontamination with quinolones and nystatin reduces gram-negative and fungal infections in orthotopic liver transplant recipients. Cleve Clin J Med 60:139-144
13. Smith SD, Jackson RJ, Hannakan CJ et al (1993) Selective decontamination in pediatric liver tranplants. Transplantation 55:1306-1309
14. Bion JF, Badger I, Crosby HA et al (1994) Selective decontamination of the digestive tract reduces Gram-negative pulmonary colonisation but not systemic endotoxemia in patients undergoing elective liver transplantation. Crit Care Med 110:303-310
15. Steffen R, Reinhartz O, Blumhardt G (1994) Bacterial and fungal colonization and infections using oral selective bowel decontamination in orthotopic liver transplantations. Transplant Int 7:101-108
16. Decruyenaere J, Colardyn F, Vogelaers D et al (1995) Combined use of fluconazole and selective digestive decontamination in the prevention of fungal infection after adult liver transplantation. Transplant Proc 27:3515-3516
17. Arnow PM, Carandang GC (1996) Randomized controlled trial of selective bowel decontamination for prevention of infections following liver transplantation. Clin Infect Dis 22:997-1003
18. Kuo PC, Bartlett ST, Lim JW et al (1997) Selective bowel decontamination in hospitalized patients awaiting liver transplantation. Am J Surg 174:745-749
19. Hjortrup A, Rasmussen A, Hansen BA et al (1997) Early bacterial and fungal infections in liver transplantation after oral selective bowel decontamination. Transplant Proc 29:3106-3110
20. Ermre S, Sebatian A, Chodoff L et al (1999) Selective decontamination of the digestive tract helps prevent bacterial infections in the early postoperative period after liver transplant. Mt Sinai J Med 66:310-313

21. Hellinger WC, Yao JD, Alvarez S et al (2002) A randomized, prospective, double-blinded evaluation of selective bowel decontamination in liver transplantation. Transplantation 73:1904-1909
22. Zwaveling JH, Maring JK, Klompmaker IJ et al (2002) Selective decontamination of the digestive tract to prevent postoperative infection: a randomized placebo-controlled trial in liver transplant patients. Crit Care Med 30:1204-1209
23. Rayes N, Seehofer D, Hansen S et al (2002) Early enteral supply of lactobacillus and fiber versus selective bowel decontamination: a controlled trial in liver transplant recipients. Transplantation 74:123-128
24. Nathens AB, Marshall JC (1999) Selective decontamination of the digestive tract in surgical patients: a systematic review of the evidence. Arch Surg 134:170-176
25. Safdar N, Said A, Lucey MR (2004) The role of selective digestive decontamination for reducing infection in patients undergoing liver transplantation: a systematic review and meta-analysis. Liver Transpl 10:817-827
26. de Jonge E, Schultz MJ, Spanjaard L et al (2003) Effects of selective decontamination of digestive tract on mortality and acquisition of resistant bacteria in intensive care: a randomised controlled trial. Lancet 362:1011-1016

Chapter 14
Do Burn Patients Benefit from Digestive Tract Decontamination?

Jacqueline E.H.M. Vet and Dave P. Mackie

Introduction

Burn injury has long been associated with infection and sepsis. In addition to the loss of function of the skin as a physical barrier, extensive burns provoke a prolonged systemic inflammatory response, with extreme fluctuations in fluid and electrolyte balance, and impairment of the immune response. Therefore, it is of the utmost importance to protect the patients affected from infections. This means that infection control is the cornerstone of good management of burn injuries. Infection prevention can be based on the pillars explained below.

Microbiological Monitoring

In-depth understanding of a patient's indigenous microbial flora is essential for preventing infection. Sources of infection can be both endogenous and exogenous (Chapter 2). In order to detect these distinct sources of infection, an initial set of cultures (throat, rectum, nose, blood, tracheal aspirate, urine, wounds) is taken on admission to the burns unit, followed by twice-weekly surveillance cultures. In addition to the standard SDD cultures from throat and rectum, specimens of urine and from the nose and wounds are also cultured twice weekly. Tracheal secretions should be taken twice weekly for culture from patients on a ventilator. Blood and catheter tip cultures are taken as indicated.

Microbiological results act as a guide for (1) determining antibiotic therapy (local and systemic), (2) initiating isolation measures if necessary, and (3) obtaining insight into the epidemiology of infection in the burns unit.

Supporting the Immune System

The pathophysiological changes that occur within the immune system after a burn injury are well documented, but the mechanisms involved are only partly understood [1, 2].

P.H.J. van der Voort, H.K.F. van Saene (eds.) *Selective Digestive Tract Decontamination in Intensive Care Medicine*. © Springer 2008

General measures designed to maintain immunocompetence include preservation of homeostasis and attenuation of the hypermetabolic response to burn injury. Patients with extensive burns loose significant amounts of fluid, electrolytes, minerals and proteins through the wounds. Adequate replacement of these losses is essential.

Preserving the integrity of the intestine by early commencement of enteral feeding [3], immunonutrition and stimulation of the microcirculation through adequate fluid maintenance (possibly assisted by vasodilators) may help to prevent translocation of endotoxins and bacteria [4–8].

It is possible to modify the (hyper-)catabolic response by avoiding energy-consuming processes, such as unnecessary stress responses caused by pain or cold [9]. Therefore, the development and implementation of sedation and pain-relief protocols are important. Patients should be nursed in an environment of relatively high warmth and humidity. Furthermore, maintenance of normoglycaemia and administration of the testosterone analogue, oxandrolon, have been shown to reduce weight loss in children and adults.

Surgical Management of Wounds

The surgical management of the patient with multiple burns is of foremost importance and is aimed primarily at swift closure of the wounds to restore the barrier function of the skin. Depending on the depth of the wound, excision and autografting are carried out, either early (3–7 days after the burn injury is sustained) or late (after two weeks), depending on the depth of injury [9, 10].

Topical Antimicrobial Therapy

The aim is to restrict microorganism colonisation of the wound to such a degree that infection is prevented. Several different types of ointments are used, and they are applied during the daily dressing changes [11–14]. The two most commonly used agents in our burn centre are silver sulphadiazine (SSD) for a total burnt skin area (TBSA) <25% and cerium silver sulphadiazine for a TBSA >25%. If wound colonisation with PPM is detected, local therapy may be switched to a more specific agent, such as silver nitrate (effective against Gram-negative microorganisms) or nitrofurazone (for *S. aureus*).

General Hygiene Precautions

The general hygiene precautions that obtain in general ICUs are imperative in the burns unit [15]. Standardisation of general procedures in a protocol helps to implement and revise these measures, examples being hand-washing and i.v. catheter care. In view of the high infection risk faced by burn patients, extra precautionary measures are taken in their care, including the use of gloves for each patient contact and the wearing of facemasks, cap and gown during dressing changes.

Isolation Procedures

Isolation is a specific precautionary measure taken with the aim of protecting the patient from colonisation from exogenous sources, including cross-infection [16]. Patients with a TBSA >25% are routinely nursed in an isolation unit equipped with a negative-pressure sluice. When the TBSA has been reduced to <25%, depending on the condition of the patient the isolation precautions may be eased. Each unit has a specified facility for disinfecting hands (alcohol dispenser) and for the disposal of contaminated material. The effectiveness of these measures is periodically checked by microbiologist and intensivist, working together to evaluate the prevalence of microbiological strains.

Selective Digestive Tract Decontamination

The aforementioned precautions do not always prevent colonisation in a patient with burn injuries. Classic studies in the 1970s showed that extreme isolation measures do reduce cross-infection but do not reduce the more frequently occurring endogenous infections [17, 18]. SDD aims to prevent colonisation from endogenous sources by eliminating Gram-negative PPM from the digestive tract by means of nonabsorbable antibiotics administered locally [19]. The anaerobic flora that contribute to colonisation resistance are selectively spared. The antibiotics are chosen specifically because they remain active in a faecal environment. Experience with the use of SDD regimens in patients with burns varies [20, 21]; our own has been very positive (Fig. 14.1) and is in line with the recent data published by de la Cal [22–24]. The SDD regimen that we use is still based on the original Groningen regimen (see Chapter 1) [19]. In a RCT, De la Cal studied 53 burn patients treated with SDD and 54 placebo controls [24]. The mortality was significantly lower in the SDD-treated patients (RR 0.28, 95%,CI 0.08–0.76), as it was for hospital mortality. The incidence of pneumonia was significantly higher in the control group. This effect was reached with the same antimicrobial combination as we use (PTA) but without intranasal mupirocin, which may explain the high incidence of staphylococcal infections in the de la Cal study [24].

Patients with a TBSA >25% and all ventilated patients (with or without inhalation trauma) are treated according to the above SDD regimen (Table 14.1). Since its introduction in 1988, we have observed a reduction in infection and mortality rates. There has been no development of resistant strains. The "search and destroy" policy of the Dutch government keeps the national incidence of MRSA between 1% and 1.5%. When MRSA is known to be present vancomycin

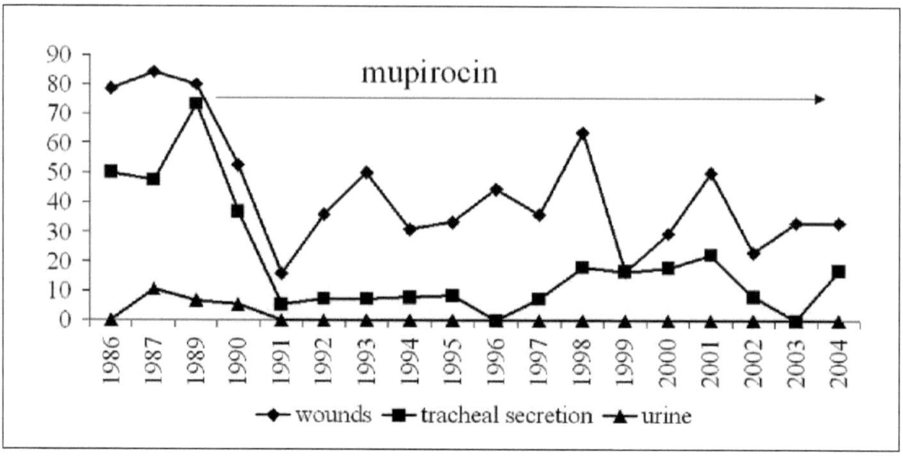

Fig. 14.1 *S. aureus* after introduction of mupirocin (% of patients colonised)

Table 14.1 Components of the SDD regimen (for more detail see Chapter 5

Four times daily orally/by nasogastric tube	First 4 days
Polymyxin E 100 mg, Tobramycin 80 mg, amphotericin B 500 mg	Cefotaxime 1 g q.i.d., i.v.
Four times daily to mouth cavity	
Polymyxin, tobramycin and amphotericin B in 2% in paste	

should be added to the preparations administered enterally and to the oral paste. This is described in Chapter 5 and also by Cerda [25].

Practical Implementation

The procedures and precautions outlined above comprise a rational approach to preventing infection and colonisation in the burns unit.

Owing to the high risk of systemic infections, colonisation (except by *Enterococci*) is not tolerated in wounds and organs. Positive wound cultures will prompt adjustment of topical wound therapy. Systemic effects (pyrexia, elevated leucocyte count) are treated by early, narrow-spectrum antibiotic therapy adjusted on the basis of the culture results.

The nature of their injuries means that most patients with burns show signs of systemic inflammatory response syndrome (SIRS) and infections can be difficult to detect. Ancillary tests, such as C-reactive protein and procalcitonin measurements, show increasing promise as aids to the diagnosis of sepsis [26]. Frank infections are always treated with systemic antibiotics.

Through the concept of SDD in combination with mupirocin in the nose (introduced in 1991 [27]), topical wound therapy and patient isolation, we have developed an infection prevention protocol that allows us to effectively decontaminate a patient by eliminating endogenous infection sources and to detect possible recontamination.

The introduction of SDD at the end of 1988 resulted in a significant reduction in colonisation and a total eradication of infections caused by Enterobacteriaceae. The major pathogen in our burns centre is *Pseudomonas*, which colonises 30% of our patients. *Pseudomonas* is responsible for predominantly exogenous wound colonisation. Only a few of these patients go on to develop an actual infection. However, *Pseudomonas* wound infection presents a continuous clinical problem: since it delays wound healing and has a negative effect on cosmetic results, the development of clinical wound sepsis with *Pseudomonas* is a serious complication, leading to systemic dysfunction and multi-organ failure (MOF). Detecting possible sources has proved difficult in practice. *Pseudomonas* was recently discovered in the sinks in the isolation units (see Fig. 14.2).

Staphylococcus aureus is found in the wounds of 40% of our patients. Wounds are gradually colonised after two weeks, but *S. aureus* is of little clinical consequence owing to the low pathogenicity and the noninvasive properties of this organism. However, there is an increased risk of pneumonia if the sputum is colonised. Figure 14.3 shows an actual colonisation of tracheal secretions. *Staphylococcus aureus* colonisation of the mouth and throat has been reduced by two thirds since we have been using SDD in combination with mupirocin. It is possible that *S. aureus* carriers are at greater risk of colonisation of their burn injuries.

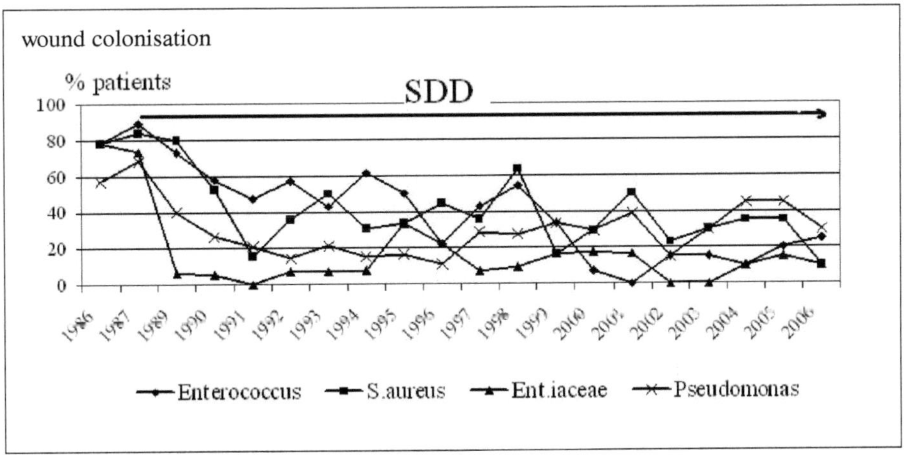

Fig. 14.2 Wound colonisation of patients with total burnt skin area (TBSA) >30% in period 1986–2006

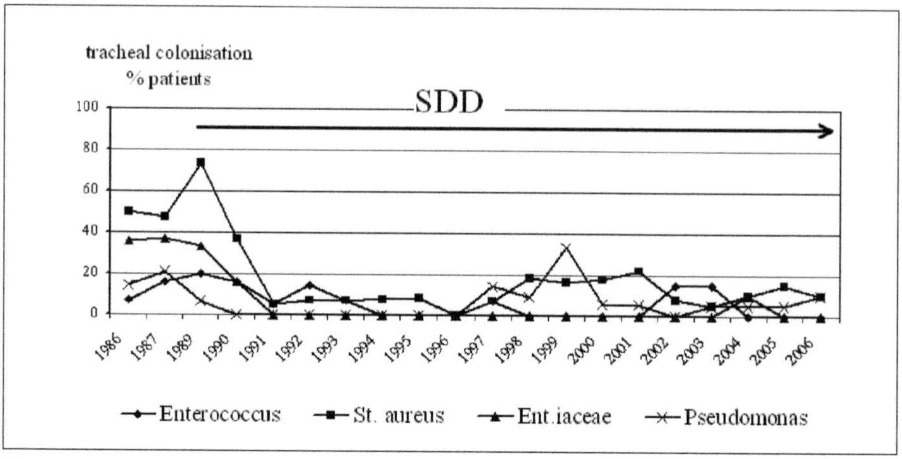

Fig. 14.3 Colonisation of tracheal secretions in patients with TBSA > 30% in period 1986–2006

Colonisation by enterococci has also declined since the 1980s. In our patient population, therefore, overgrowth of enterococci has not been observed to result from use of the SDD regimen. In general enterococci do not cause clinical infection, although positive blood cultures have been found in patients already compromised by sepsis due to another organism.

Intravenous catheter sepsis is rarely seen, owing to our current protocol, which involves changing catheters every seven days. However, between 1999 and 2004, there were seven proven cases of "line sepsis" caused by a central venous catheter, four infected with an enterococcus and three, with *S. epidermidis*. These infections had minimal clinical consequences. It is possible that these recent incidents suggest a change in the virulence of enterococci, as suggested elsewhere. There is no evidence that the resistance pattern of enterococcus has changed in our unit since we started using SDD.

Fungal infections are virtually unknown in our burn centre, possibly due to the use of amphotericin B in the orabase and SDD suspension [28].

Our data indicate that, since the introduction of SDD in combination with mupirocin, there has been a significant reduction in mortality and in the rates of pneumonia, sepsis and wound infections. At the same time, there is little or no evidence of resistant Gram-negative strains. Consequently, since the introduction of SDD in 1987, there have been no closures of the burns unit because of multi-resistant aerobic Gram-negative bacteria.

It has to be emphasised that, in addition to the SDD regimen, we adhere strictly to conventional infection prevention protocols. Good cooperation between the medical microbiologist, hygienist, and nurses and doctors ensures adequate implementation of the SDD protocol.

Our actual mortality rate during the period of 1988 to 2005 has been extremely low. In comparison with the Bull and Fisher mortality chart recently updated by Rashid (see Fig. 14.4) [29], we see a mortality rate of 8% in patients with large burn injuries, as against a predicted mortality of 21%. The main cause of mortality in our burns unit is now (multi)organ failure caused by the patho-physiological challenge posed by extensive burn injury, aggravated by pre-existing co-morbidity, but without symptoms of infection. Our experience suggests that our current policy has led to effective control of infection and relatively low mortality in the burns unit (see Fig. 14.5).

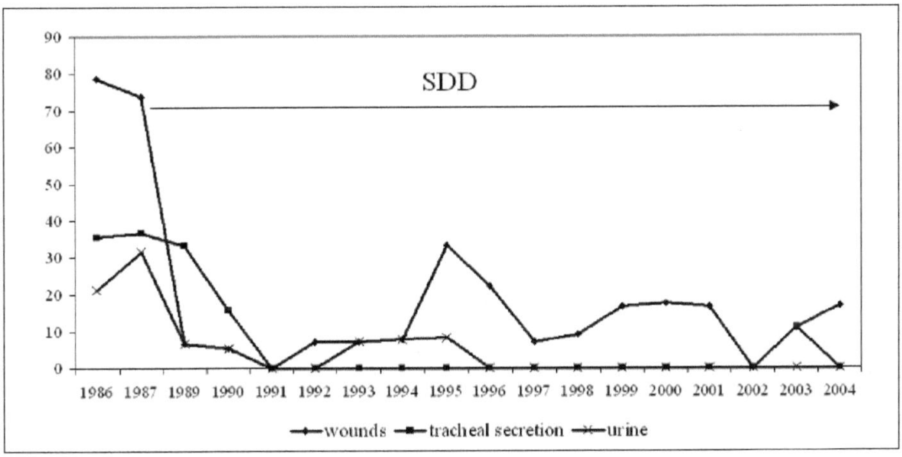

Fig 14.4 Effect of SDD on colonisation AGNB (% of patients colonised)

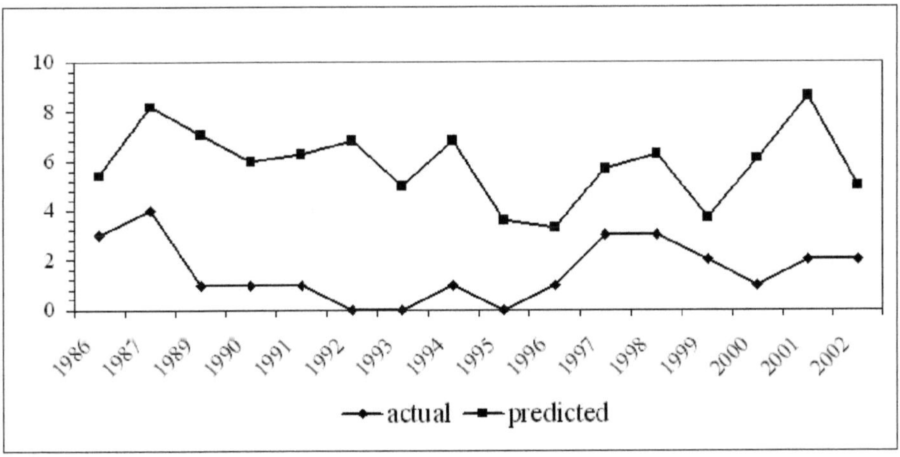

Fig. 14.5 Actual mortality of patients with TBSA >30% in period 1986–2002 compared with predicted mortality (Rashid et al. [29]).

Conclusion

All data show that severely burned patients benefit from SDD (PTA topically and cefotaxime i.v.) in terms of infection prevention and mortality. The addition of intranasal mupirocine appears to have controlled staphylococcal pneumonia. No multi-resistant strains have emerged during 18 years' experience with SDD in our burns centre.

References

1. Warden GD (1987) Immunological alterations following thermal injury. In Achauer B (ed) Management of the burn patient. Appleton & Lang, Norwalk, Conn.
2. Gibran NS, Heimbach DM (1993) Mediators in thermal injury. Semin Nephrol 13:344-358
3. Klasen HJ, ten Duis HJ (1987) Early oral feeding of patients with extensive burns. Burns 13:49-52
4. Zielger TR, Smith RJ, O'Dwyer ST, et al (1988) Increased intestinal permeability associated with infection in burn patients. Arch Surg 123:1459-1464
5. Desai MH, Herndon DN, Rutan RL, et al (1991) Ischemic intestinal complications in patients with burns. Surg Gynecol Obstet 172:257-261
6. Deitch EA (1990) Intestinal permeability is increased in burn patients shortly after injury. Surgery 107:411-416
7. Wilmore DW, Smith RJ, O'Dwyer ST, et al (1988) The gut: a central organ after surgical stress. Surgery 104:917-923
8. Deitch EA, Winterton J, Berg RB (1987) The gut as a portal of entry for bacteremia: role of protein malnutrition. Ann Surg 205:681-692
9. Dobke MK, Simoni J, Ninnemann JL, et al (1989) Endotoxemia after burn injury: effect of early excision on circulating endotoxin levels. J Burn Care Rehabil 10:107-111
10. Order SE, Mason AD, Walker HL, et al (1965) The pathogenesis of second and third degree burns and conversion to full thickness injury. Surg Gynecol Obstet 120:983-991
11. Lindberg RB, Moncrief JA, Mason AD (1968) Control of experimental and clinical burn wound sepsis by topical application of sulfamylon compounds. Ann N Y Acad Sci 150:950-960
12. Moyer CA, Brentano L, Gravens D, et al (1965) Treatment of large human burns with 0.5% silver nitrate solution. Arch Surg 91:812-817
13. Fox CL (1968) Silver sulfadiazine—a new topical therapy for Pseudomonas in burns. Arch Surg 96:185-188
14. Hermans RP, Schumburg T (1982) Silver sulfadiazine versus silver sulfadiazine—cerium nitrate. Abstracts of the 6th I.S.B.I. Congress, San Francisco
15. McManus AT, McManus WF, Mason AD Jr, et al (1985) Microbial colonization in a new intensive care burn unit. A prospective cohort study. Arch Surg 120:217-223
16. Lee JJ, Marvin JA, Heimbach DM, et al (1990) Infection control in a burns centre. J Burn Care Rehabil 11:575-580
17. Lowbury EJL, Babb JR, Ford PM (1971) Protective isolation in a burns unit: the use of plastic isolators and air curtains. J Hyg 69:529-546
18. Burke JF, Quimby WC, Bondoc CC, et al (1977) The contribution of a bacterially isolated environment to the prevention of infection in seriously burned patients. Ann Surg 186:377-387
19. Stoutenbeek CP, van Saene HKF, Miranda DR, et al (1984) The effect of selective decontamination of the digestive tract on colonisation and infection rate in multiple trauma patients. Intensive Care Med 10:185-192
20. Barret JP, Jeschke MG, Herden DN (2001) Selective decontamination of the digestive tract in severely burned pediatric patients. Burns 27:439-445

21. Manson WL, Klasen HJ, Sauer EW, et al (1992) Selective intestinal decontamination for prevention of wound colonisation in severely burned patients: a retrospective analysis. Burns 18:98-102
22. Mackie DP, van Hertum WAJ, Schumburg T, et al (1992) Prevention of infection in burns: preliminary experience with selective decontamination of the digestive tract in patients with extensive injuries. J Trauma 32:570-575
23. Mackie DP, van Hertum WAJ (1998) El control de la infección en los quemados. In: Lorente JA, Esteban A (eds) Cuidados intensivos del patiente quemado. Springer-Verlag Iberia, Barcelona New York London
24. de la Cal MA, Cerda E, Garcia-Hierro P, van Saene HK, et al (2005) Survival benefit in critically ill burned patients receiving selective decontamination of the digestive tract: a randomized, placebo-controlled, double-blind trial. Ann Surg 241:424-430
25. Cerda E, Abella A, de la Cal MA, et al (2007) Enteral vancomycin controls methicillin-resistant Staphylococcus aureus endemicity in an intensive care burn unit. A 9-year prospective study. Ann Surg 245:397-407
26. Lavrentieva A, Kontakiotis T, Lazaridis L, et al (2007) Inflammatory markers in patients with severe burn injury. What is the best indicator of sepsis? Burns 33:189-194
27. Mackie DP, van Hertum WAJ, Schumburg T, et al (1994) Staphylococcus aureus wound colonisation following the addition of methylmupirocine to a regimen of selective decontamination in extensive burns. Burns 20/1:14-18
28. Silvestri L, van Saene HKF, Milanese M, et al (2007) Selective decontamination of the digestive tract reduces bacterial bloodstream infection and mortality in critically ill patients. Systematic review of randomised, controlled trials. J Hosp Infect 65:187-203
29. Rashid A, Khanna A, Gowar JP, Bull JP (2001) Revised estimates of mortality from burns in the last 20 years at the Birmingham Burns Centre. Burns 27:723-730

Chapter 15
How to Design an Antibiotic Strategy That Respects the Indigenous Flora

Hans L. Bams

Introduction

This chapter is meant to give practical guidelines on developing an antibiotic policy, bearing in mind the philosophy and goals [1] of selective decontamination of the digestive tract (SDD) as described in the earlier chapters of this book. These guidelines may be needed because SDD is meant to change the resident flora in such a way that secondary endogenous infections by that flora will not occur. As antibiotics given for (suspected) infection usually affect the resident flora, these antibiotics can easily interact in such a way as to conflict with the aims of SDD. Antibiotics can interact in several ways. They can inactivate the topical antibiotics used to achieve SDD, and they can also interact with the colonisation resistance. These guidelines will give some help in the choice of an antibiotic therapy that will allow both goals to be achieved: eliminating infection and persistence of colonisation resistance by unaffected gut flora with anaerobes and Gram-positive bacilli.

SDD is most effective when the full SDD protocol is used: topical antibiotics in the gastrointestinal tract combined with a 4-day course of a specific i.v. antibiotic. This chapter will deal with the choice of both the i.v. antibiotic for the 4-day course and any additional antibiotics when these are needed during SDD for treatment of infections. In the latter situation a distinction can be made between decontaminated patients and patients who have not yet been decontaminated. Patients can be considered decontaminated when they have passed stools while on SDD for at least two days. The ultimate proof of decontamination is when the stool culture shows no growth of potential pathogenic microorganisms (PPM), and in particular of aerobic Gram-negative bacteria (AGNB).

Criteria for Antibiotic Choice

Selective decontamination of the digestive tract (SDD) in critically ill patients aims at *selective* elimination of the AGNB and yeasts from the alimentary tract whilst the anaerobic flora remains unaffected. This means that, whenever additional i.v. antibiotics need to be prescribed, they also have to meet these criteria. Additionally prescribed antibiotics, therefore, need to meet the following demands (see also earlier chapters describing the basics of SDD):

1 No interference with colonisation pattern/resistance in the alimentary tract, e.g. nonpathogenic and the anaerobic microorganisms left unaffected;
2 Low risk of emerging antibiotic resistance, especially resistance to the antibiotics contained in the SDD medication;
3 Anti-inflammatory propensities.

Interference with colonisation resistance. All antibiotics that are active against other bacteria than AGNB or yeasts interfere with the colonisation resistance. The disappearance of AGNB from the digestive tract gives rise to an increase in other aerobic bacteria, such as enterococci. When antibiotics that are active against enterococci are used, other aerobic bacteria might be able to colonise the gut. The antibiotics that are most harmful in this context are all penicillin-derived antibiotics, including imipenem and meronem. Co-trimoxazole has a limited effect on colonisation resistance and can be used occasionally. However, for some Gram-positive infections it may be necessary to use, as briefly as possible, such antibiotics as clindamycin or vancomycin.

Ceftriaxon (Rocephin®) impairs colonisation resistance by inactivating the tobramycin in the SDD through the enterohepatic cycle and excretion via bile into the digestive tract [2]. As cefotaxime is not characterised by bile excretion, this interaction will not occur during i.v. treatment with cefotaxime. Amoxicillin/clavulanic acid (Augmentin®) inactivates the SDD through the clavulanic acid [3]. In addition, amoxicillin interferes with the colonisation resistance by its action on the anaerobic flora.

As already stated, ideally the parenteral component of SDD respects the patient's gut ecology. However, in certain circumstances the parenteral component may affect the anaerobes. Fortunately, the enteral antimicrobials control overgrowth of AGNB and yeasts and they control a possible side effect of disregard for the patients gut ecology.

Low resistance potential. In general, the first infections with microorganisms resistant to a new anti-microbial agent emerge 2 years after the launch of the new antibiotic. For example, linezolid was promoted on the market for clinical practice in 2000, and in 2002 the first reports of MRSA resistant to linezolid were published. We have used antimicrobials with low resistance potential, i.e. older agents that are still active after several years. For example, the first-generation cephalosporins, cefazolin and cephradin, are still active against *Staphylococcus aureus*. To give another example, the enteral component of SDD, polymyxin, is still active against most AGNBs 50 years after the onset of clinical use. This major difference between high resistance potential and low resistance potential is due to mechanism of action of the antimicrobial and its pharmacokinetics. Polymyxins interfere with cell wall synthesis, and cephazolin and cephradin do not impact on gut flora in selecting resistant mutants amongst gut bacteria. Amoxicillin is very sensitive to beta-lactamases and promotes overgrowth of gut AGNB owing to interference with the colonisation resistance.

Anti-inflammatory propensities. All beta-lactams and fluoroquinolones are unable to inactivate endotoxins released following the killing of sensitive microorganisms. These antimicrobials have been shown to promote the release of cytokines and subsequently the inflammatory state of the patient. Glycopeptides, aminoglycosides, polyenes and polymyxins have recently been shown to possess anti-inflammatory characteristics [4].

During the development of the SDD protocol these three important criteria were taken into account in the choice of the decontaminating agents. For topical decontamination, the optimal combination appeared to be polymyxin E, tobramycin and amphotericin B (see Chapter 1). We have used these antibiotics in our SDD protocol for more than twenty years. Overgrowth of potentially pathogenic microorganisms has not occurred to a degree that it could have led to an outbreak of superinfections. As a consequence, the intensive care unit has never been closed because of an epidemic caused by multi-resistant bacteria. Apparently, the addition of enteral antimicrobials to the parenteral agents is crucial in the control of overgrowth of PPMs, and probably in the prevention of resistance (see also Chapter 9). The enteral antimicrobials prevent the emergence of resistance mutants amongst the gut flora, which means these older parenteral agents are still useful.

These considerations have led to the following antibiotic protocol.

Antibiotic Protocol for ICU Patients With Infection Who Will Also Be Treated With SDD

Introduction

The most common sites of infection in critically ill patients are:

- Lower airways
- Blood
- Abdomen
- Invasive foreign bodies, such as CVP lines, Swan-Ganz catheters, drains
- Wounds
- Bladder
- Sinuses

Microbiological sampling to confirm an infection needs diagnostic samples of blood, tracheal aspirate, urine, etc., which are taken as clinically indicated. In contrast, surveillance samples to detect the abnormal carrier state are taken on admission and then routinely twice weekly, for instance, on Mondays and Thursdays (see Chapter 4).

Antibiotic Strategies: the 4-Day i.v. Antibiotic Course

The standard 4-day i.v. antibiotic course at the start of SDD is cefotaxime 1,000 mgr 4 times daily i.v. for 96 hours. This systemic administration is mandatory because SDD takes 2–4 days to become effective in critically ill patients owing to motility dysfunction of the gastrointestinal tract. In addition, cefotaxime will treat primary endogenous infections that are active at the time of the start of SDD (usually on admission to the ICU). The choice of cefotaxime over other i.v. antibiotics is based on the criteria mentioned above (colonisation resistance, low resistance potential and anti-inflammatory propensities) and also on the anticipated PPMs that may be present in the airways or other potentially infected site. It is mandatory to look for previous microbiological results taken at previous admissions or during previous infections. These samples can inform us about the carrier status and the microorganisms that we can expect during the current admission. Depending on this information, other i.v. antibiotics can be added to cefotaxime.

Antimicrobial Therapy in Sepsis–microorganism and Source Not Known

In general, three syndromes are distinguished: pneumosepsis, urosepsis and abdominal sepsis (Table 15.1).

Pneumosepsis

1. Community-acquired pneumosepsis: Cefotaxime combined with erythromycin to cover community microorganisms and atypical microorganisms such as *Legionella pneumophila*. Ciprofloxacin is an alternative to erythromycin.
2. Hospital-acquired pneumosepsis: Cefotaxime combined with ciprofloxacin to cover both community and hospital bacteria. Aminoglycosides are best avoided because a high percentage of critically ill patients have impaired renal function and are at risk of acute renal failure. Aminoglycosides are potentially nephrotoxic and can increase the incidence of acute renal failure. The basic strategy is to eliminate abnormal carriage and pathologic colonisation. In the case of lower airway infection, abnormal carriage should be elim-

Table 15.1 Antimicrobial therapy in sepsis–microorganism and source NOT known (CAP, community-acquired pneumosepsis; HAP, hospital-acquired pneumosepsis)

Pneumosepsis	CAP	Cefotaxim with erythromycin or ciprofloxacin
	HAP	Cefotaxim with ciprofloxacin
Urosepsis		Cefotaxim with ciprofloxacin
Abdominal sepsis		Cefotaxim with ciprofloxacin, metronidazol and amphotericin B

inated by nebulised antibiotics. Gram-negative bacteria can be treated by aerosolised tobramycin (40 or 80 mg q.i.d.) or polymyxin E (5 ml of a 2% solution q.i.d.). *Staphylococcus aureus* can be eliminated by aerosolised cefotaxime or a first-generation cephalosporin (500 mg q.i.d.). The respiratory filter can be occluded by these antimicrobials and should be replaced after each nebulisation. Aerosolised amphotericin B (5 mg in 5 ml q.i.d.) can be used for *Candida* colonisation.

Urosepsis

Cefotaxime combined with ciprofloxacin as part of SDD prophylaxis and to eradicate AGNB from the upper and lower urinary tract. Information on previous cultures and colonisation is important. If necessary, ciprofloxacin can be replaced by other nonpenicillin antibiotics, such as co-trimoxazole.

Abdominal Sepsis

Cefotaxime combined with ciprofloxacin, metronidazol and amphotericin B to cover AGNB, anaerobes and yeasts.

In addition, all patients receive the full four-component of SDD to prevent secondary endogenous and exogenous infection with ICU-associated microorganisms.

Antimicrobial Therapy in Sepsis–microorganism or Source Known (Table 15.2)

Table 15.2 Antimicrobial therapy in sepsis–microorganism OR source known (AGNB, aerobic Gram-negative bacteria)

Organ	Microorganism	Antibiotic(s)
Lungs	AGNB	Cefotaxim[a]
	AGNB unknown	Ciprofloxacin + tobramycin
	AGNB in tracheal aspirate	Aerosol of tobramycin or polymyxin
	Enterococci	Amoxicillin
Urinary tract[b]	Enterococci	Amoxicillin 3 doses
	AGNB	Cefotaxim or ciprofloxacin
	Yeasts	5 mg amphotericin B in 100 ml solution 2 td for two days in the bladder
Abdomen	Nondecontaminated patient	Cefotaxim + ciprofloxacin + metronidazol
	Decontaminated patient	Amoxicillin 5 days
Intravasal lines[c]	Vancomycin 2 td 1 g for 2 days	

[a]For AGNB in lungs: in case of *Serratia* spp., *Pseudomonas* spp. and *Acinetobacter* spp., ciprofloxacin is preferred to cefotaxim. For *Stenotrophomonas* spp. co-trimoxazole is preferred. [b]Urinary catheter should be changed before second antibiotic dose. [c]Change line after first dose

Lungs

Check previous cultures! In the case of AGNB use a cephalosporin (cefotaxime) whenever possible. For *Serratia* spp., *Pseudomonas* spp., *Stenotrophomonas* spp. and *Acinetobacter* spp., ciprofloxacin is preferred. When the type of AGNB is unknown, ciprofloxacin should be given together (or combined) with a single dose of tobramycin of 4 mg/kg i.v. The dose of tobramycin needs to be adjusted to kidney function. In the case of AGNB in tracheal aspirate or bronchoalveolar lavage, fluid aerosolised tobramycin (80 mg q.i.d.) or polymyxin 2% 5 ml four times daily may be aerosolised to the lungs. In some cases cefotaxime 500 mg aerosolised q.i.d. may be preferred. The i.v. tobramycin should be administered for the shortest period possible owing to the narrow therapeutic range and the risk of renal failure in multiple organ failure patients. In the case of enterococci: check for enterococci faecium because of amoxicillin resistance. All amoxycillin-sensitive strains can be treated with amoxycillin for a maximum of five days. One should be reluctant to treat enterocci in the respiratory tract, as they can mostly be regarded as colonisation.

Urinary tract

Urinary cultures are usually not routinely performed during SDD. Therefore, the suspicion of a urinary tract infection should prompt a new urinary culture. When patients are adequately decontaminated (confirmed by stool surveillance culture) the most probable bacteria are enterococci. Therefore, a short course of three doses of amoxycillin is enough to treat a urinary tract infection with enterococci, providing the urinary catheter is removed and replaced between the first and second doses. For AGNB urinary infection cefotaxime or ciproxin is preferred. Occasionally yeast infection of the urinary tract occurs. This can be treated by four doses (two days) of 100 ml of a solution containing 5 mg of amphotericin B. This solution can be instilled into the bladder and followed by closing of the urinary catheter for 1–2 hours. After two doses of amphotericin B the urinary catheter should be replaced.

Abdomen

Patients admitted to the ICU with perforation of the gut and peritonitis should receive the full SDD protocol in addition to a course of other antibiotics. To complete the Gram-negative spectrum of cefotaxime, we advise administration of ciprofloxacin or tobramycin i.v.; Ciprofloxacin is preferred because of its wider therapeutic range and better penetration. Metronidazol should also be added for a short period of time. As most people are colonised with yeasts in the digestive tract (both upper and lower), it is advisable to add antifungal therapy until the culture results are available. Within 3–4 days it should be clear which bacteria are present in the abdomen, and the regimen can then be restricted.

When a gut perforation occurs during SDD in a patient who has been decontaminated, only enterococci and anaerobes enter the abdominal space. The peritonitis is usually mild, and a limited course of amoxicillin (five days) in addition to the surgical treatment is usually enough.

Intravasal lines as possible cause.

Vancomycin 1 g once or twice daily i.v. for two days and, obviously, removal of the line responsible.

Antimicrobial Therapy in the Presence of Endocarditis–source Not Known

Acute endocarditis. First-generation cephalosporin 2 g i.v. six times daily and gentamicin one dose of 4 mg/kg. Duration of therapy: guided by clinical picture and based on CRP.
Subacute/chronic endocarditis. Vancomycin 1 g i.v. once or twice daily plus gentamicin one dose of 4 mg/kg whenever artificial material (valve, patch, etc.) is present. If there is no artificial material, amoxicillin 1 g four times daily g i.v. plus gentamicin in one dose of 4 mg/kg (Table 15.3).

Antimicrobial Therapy in the Case of Endocarditis–source Known

In the case of endocarditis demonstrably caused by coagulase-negative streptococci (CNS), vancomycin 2 td 1 g i.v. for a minimum of six weeks, rifampin 3 td 300 mg i.v. guided by CRP and gentamicin one dose of 4 mg/kg i.v. for two weeks (Table 15.3).

Antimicrobial Therapy in the Case of Sinusitis–source Not Known

Co-trimoxazol 2 td 960 mg i.v. Can be extended by addition of metronidazol 3 td 500 mg i.v.

When sinusitis occurs during ICU treatment enterococci are the most frequent bacteria, and it should thus be treated with amoxicillin i.v. In all situations drainage of the sinus should be performed.

Table 15.3 Antimicrobial therapy in endocarditis (CNS, coagulase-negative streptococci)

Source NOT known	Acute endocarditis	First-generation cephalosporin 6 td 2 g and gentamicin 1 dose of 4 mg/kg
	Subacute/chronic endocarditis	Vancomycin 2 td 1 g and gentamicin 1 dose of 4 mg/kg in presence of artificial material Amoxicillin 4 td 1 g plus gentamicin 1 dose of 4 mg/kg if NO artificial material present
Source KNOWN	Acute endocarditis caused by CNS	Vancomycin 2 td 1 g for at least 6 weeks + rifampicin 3 td 300 mg (guided by CRP) and gentamicin 1 dose of 4 mg/kg in 2 weeks

Antimicrobial Therapy in the Case of Pneumonia–source Not Known

See under Antimicrobial therapy in sepsis–pneumosepsis

Antimicrobial Therapy in the Case of Confirmed Aspiration

When aspiration occurs under SDD, enterococci are the expected microorganisms. As these bacteria show a low pathogenicity this situation usually does *not* need antibiotic treatment. If antibiotics are needed, amoxicillin i.v. should be given.

Antimicrobial Therapy in the Case of Urinary Tract Infection–source Not Known

Ciprofloxacin 2 td 200 mg i.v. When enterococci are suspected as a possible cause (under SDD): amoxicillin 4 td 1 g i.v.

In the case of yeasts: see Antimicrobial therapy in sepsis–Source known: Urinary tract.

Antimicrobial Therapy in Case of Mediastinitis–Source Not Known

Vancomycin i.v., guided by blood levels

In the case of *S. aureus* a first-generation cephalosporin is adequate and does not interfere with the colonisation resistance.

The therapy should be continued until at least two negative cultures have been obtained.

Antimicrobial Therapy in Case of Yeasts

Yeast in sputum: 4 td 5 mg amphotericin B by aerosol

When after one week of SDD yeasts are still cultured from the throat, the oral dosage of SDD medications is increased to 8 td.

When invasive yeast or fungal infection is suspected, amphotericin-B is given i.v. (0.5–1.0 mg/day in a continuous infusion) or the liposomal version, e.g. ambisome is used (3–5 mg/kg per day). To obtain amphotericin B levels above MIC values for *Candida* in the peritoneal fluid, a minimum serum level of 0.5 mg/l is needed [5].

In the case of yeast in the urine: rinse the bladder with 2 td 5 mg amphotericin B diluted in 50 ml and leave it in the bladder for one hour. After the second rinse, change the urinary catheter. Duration of therapy: two days, unless otherwise indicated.

The newer antifungals can also be used. However, interaction with other drugs via the CYP 450 enzyme system is frequent. Voriconazole is the preferred drug for *Aspergillus* infections. *Aspergillus* colonisation in the airways can be treated with amphotericin B aerosol 4 td 5 mg in 5 ml.

Systemic Infection with **Pseudomonas spp**

Drugs that can be used while respecting the SDD philosophy are ciprofloxacin i.v. 2 td 200–400 mg or ceftazidim, with or without tobramycin.

With respect to the use of SDD: try to avoid piperacillin, meropenem and imipenem because of their effects on colonisation resistance.

Systemic Infection with **Enterococci**

Amoxicillin 4 td 1 g i.v.

Systemic Infection With **Staphylococcus Epidermidis** *(CNS)*

Vancomycin 1–2 td 1 g i.v., guided by blood levels.

When antibiotics are given by aerosol they need to be continued until there have been at least two negative sputum cultures; this means that when cultures are taken twice a week this treatment will last at least ten days. It may be advisable to culture three times a week in these cases, to avoid overtreatment.

Obviously antibiotics should not be started until after the necessary cultures have been taken from the suspected sources and the blood. If blood cultures are done, it is mandatory that fresh blood taken by sterile venous punctures is used.

Suspected Infection in a Decontaminated Patient

The presentation of infection in decontaminated patients will generally be less fulminant, and infection should be suspected in the case of persistent (low-grade) fever, mild elevation of C-reactive protein and a sustained need for inotropes. By definition, patients thus affected are suffering from infection with anaerobic or Gram-positive pathogens (enterococci or CNS). The intrinsic pathogenicity index (IPI) of these microbes is low, and the inflammatory response is limited. One should therefore be reluctant to treat these infections with systemic antibiotics because additional antibiotics can interfere with colonisation resistance. For suspected enterococcal infection amoxicillin (1 g i.v. q.i.d.) should be used for a maximum of five days. For suspected CNS infection vancomycin (1–2 g per day, guided by serum levels) should be given. When amoxicillin-resistant enterococci have been identified, vancomycin should be used instead of amoxicillin. Vancomycin-resistant enterococci are usually sensitive to amoxicillin. Otherwise, the newer linezolid may be used.

This proposed antibiotic scheme is a guideline and should be treated as such. It is important to note the following remarks, regardless of which protocol is going to be used:

- Antibiotic therapy started when the source of infection is not known needs to be adjusted as soon as the source is known. The effect(s) of the necessary antibiotic on what can be achieved with SDD must be borne in mind.
- When fever persists for more than 48 hours of antibiotic therapy without manifest infection, reconsider the antibiotic selected or discontinue the antibiotic therapy and take more cultures 24–48 hours later.
- It is advisable to treat patients who have an intravenous/arterial access in the groin with SDD enemas or suppositories twice daily until rectal swabs confirm adequate decontamination and the patient passes stools as a sign of normal gastrointestinal function. The SDD enemas or suppositories contain half the oral dosages of polymyxin, tobramycin and amphotericin B.

- When SDD is being administered, twice weekly culturing of sputum, throat, urine and rectum is mandatory, as discussed in previous chapters.

Once again, all antibiotic strategies discussed in this chapter must be seen as guidelines that should be adapted to the local situation according to resistance patterns of prevalent microorganisms. However, the basic strategy with the four pillars of SDD should always be applied, and the i.v. antibiotics chosen should be those that interfere the least with this strategy.

References

1. Stoutenbeek CP (1987) Infection prevention in multiple trauma patients by selective decontamination of the digestive tract. Thesis, ISBN 90-9001736-4
2. Giamarellou H (1980) Aminoglycosides plus beta-lactams against Gram-negative organisms. Evaluation of in vitro synergy and chemical interactions. Am J Med 80(6B):126-137
3. Flournoy DJ (1979) Factors influencing the inactivation of aminoglycosides by beta-lactams. Methods Find Exp Clin Pharmacol 1:233-238
4. Holtzheimer RG (2001) Antibiotic induced endotoxin release and clinical sepsis: a review. J Chemother 13:159-172
5. Van der Voort PH, Boerma EC, Yska JP (2007) Serum and peritoneal levels of amphotericin B and flucytosine during intravenous treatment of critically ill patients with Candida peritonitis. J Antimicrob Chemother 59:952-956

Two Clinical Cases

Peter H.J. van der Voort

Case 1

A 67-year-old-man was admitted to the ICU with abdominal sepsis. A week before, he had undergone right-sided hemicolectomy. A revision operation was performed because of a rise in CRP level and abdominal pain. The ileo-colostomy appeared to be insufficient, with faecal spill into the abdominal cavity. An ileostoma was made and the colon closed. After this operation he was transferred to the ICU because of an inflammatory response with hypotension, fever and hypoxia.

1. What cultures should be taken on ICU admission?
2. How can the digestive tract of this patient be decontaminated?
3. What systemic antimicrobial agents should be used?

The tracheal aspirate appeared to grow *Pseudomonas aeruginosa* 100 colonies.

4. How can this PPM be eliminated?

The throat culture showed *Candida albicans* and *Pseudomonas aeruginosa*. The rectal swab showed *Candida albicans*, *E. coli* and *Proteus mirabilis*. The clinical course was prolonged. After two weeks, a tracheostomy was made and a duodenal tube was placed to allow full enteral nutrition.

5. What should now be changed in the decontamination policy?

After four weeks the surveillance cultures of the throat still repeatedly showed *Candida* species.

6. What three interventions would now be appropriate?

The tracheal aspirate showed Gram-positive flora for more than two weeks (which should not be treated) but now *Pseudomonas aeruginosa* was also present.

7. Was this primary endogenous/secondary endogenous/exogenous?
8. How should it be treated?

A third operation was necessary; perforation of the proximal duodenum was found.

9. Should the SDD suspension be stopped?

Case 2

A 58-year-old woman was admitted to the hospital with COPD. After two weeks her condition deteriorated, with hypercapnic respiratory failure. She was treated with amoxicillin-clavulanic acid for ten days. A new infiltrate was now seen in the right lower lobe on the chest X-ray. She was admitted to the ICU for mechanical ventilation.

1. What antimicrobial agents would be appropriate?
2. How should *Candida* colonisation in the lower airways be treated?
3. The urine contained *E. coli*. What should be done about this?

After seven days there had still been no defaecation and the rectal swabs still showed *E. coli* 3+, *Candida* and *Xanthomonas* 2+.

4. How could decontamination be promoted?
5. How could *Xanthomonas* be eliminated when this microorganism persists even after defaecation?

If MRSA were present on admission in the rectal swab:

6. How could this patient be decontaminated?

Discussion

Case 1

1. Surveillance samples: throat and rectum.
   Diagnostic samples: tracheal aspirate, urine, abdominal fluid (during operation or from the abdominal drains)
2. Oral paste with 2% PTA 4 times daily, PTA suspension 4 times daily in nasogastric tube. The ileostomy will be decontaminated when the SDD suspension passes through the digestive tract. In the meantime, some experts suggest using a suppository in the stoma. The colon, which is still in situ, can be decontaminated by rectal suppositories or enemas.
3. Antimicrobials that respect the indigenous flora must be used. For instance, the combination of cefotaxime, ciprofloxacin and metronidazole. In particular, metronidazole should be used for the shortest as possible time (e.g. five days). To eliminate enterococci, amoxicillin may be used in addition, also for the shortest possible time. Early treatment of *Candida* may be indicated, but this decision is not a part of the SDD concept.
4. Aerosolised tobramycin 4 times daily 40 or 80 mg or polymyxin 2% 5 ml four times daily. Don't forget to change the filter of the ventilator after each treatment.
5. SDD oral paste should be applied around the tracheostomy. The 10 ml sus-

pension given in the nasogastric tube should be divided into 5 ml in the nasogastric tube and 5 ml in the duodenal tube.

6. A. Check whether the oral paste is applied properly. B. Renew the gastric and duodenal tubes as they can be contaminated with *Candida* and will not be cleaned properly by the SDD paste and suspension. C. Apply the SDD oral paste 8 times a day until two consecutive cultures show no growth of *Candida*.
7. As *Pseudomonas* was found before, it is most likely the same microorganism. As such this colonisation is a primary endogenous one that has not been eliminated properly.
8. Repeat the aerosol tobramycin or polymyxin. If tobramycin was used previously, we advise using polymyxin now and vice versa.
9. Try to have a feeding tube distal to the perforation and continue to give SDD suspension by that tube. The oral paste will probably be enough to decontaminate oral, oesophageal and gastric sites, but a reduced volume of SDD suspension can be given into the stomach.

Case 2

1. The choice of the antimicrobials depends on previous cultures and local frequently found hospital flora. Try to use antimicrobials that respect the indigenous flora. Gram-negative microorganisms are very probably present, as this patient has been pretreated and has been in the hospital for two weeks. In this situation we prefer the combination of cefotaxime and ciprofloxacin.
2. *Candida* colonisation in the lower airways can be treated by amphotericin B aerosol 4 times daily, 5 mg in 5 ml. Change the filter of the ventilator after each treatment.
3. Treatment with cefotaxime and ciprofloxacin will probably be successful. However, change the urinary catheter to eliminate recolonisation of the urine. In the decontaminated patient, the urine should then stay sterile. If enterococci appear in the urine, two doses of amoxicillin 1 g should be enough, and the urinary catheter should be changed between the two doses.
4. High-dose polyethylene glycol-based laxatives or neostigmine by continuous infusion 10-20 mg per day
5. In the case of low-level growth (fewer than 1,000 colonies) it may be accepted. Otherwise it is overgrowth, with the possibility of infection, emergence of resistance or outbreak. Co-trimoxazole by nasogastric tube can be added twice daily 960 mg.
6. Add vancomycin 4 times daily 0.5 g to the SDD suspension and add vancomycin to the oral paste (Chapter 5). If the tracheal aspirate contains MRSA, vancomycin 0.25 g can be given by aerosol four times daily. Mupirocin gel can be applied in the nose. In the case of infection, vancomycin can be given i.v.

Subject Index

MIX
Papier aus verantwortungsvollen Quellen
Paper from responsible sources
FSC® C105338

If you have any concerns about our products,
you can contact us on
ProductSafety@springernature.com

In case Publisher is established outside the EU,
the EU authorized representative is:
Springer Nature Customer Service Center GmbH
Europaplatz 3, 69115 Heidelberg, Germany

Printed by Libri Plureos GmbH
in Hamburg, Germany